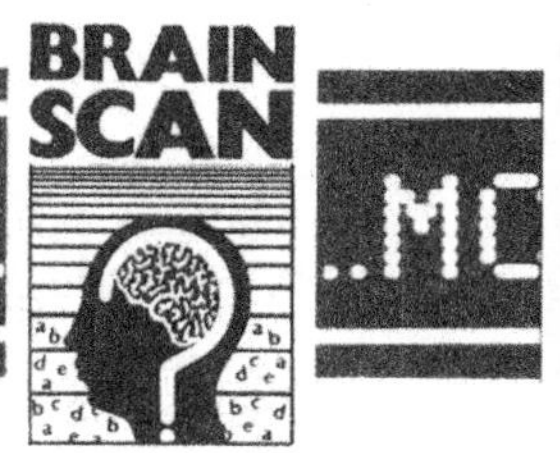

David Goldmeier · Simon Barton

Sexually Transmitted Diseases

Springer-Verlag
London Berlin Heidelberg New York
Paris Tokyo

David Goldmeier, MD, MRCP, Consultant Venereologist, St Mary's Hospital, London, W2

Simon Barton, BSc, MB, BS, Research Fellow, St Mary's Hospital, London, W2

Publishers note: the 'Brainscan' logo is reproduced by courtesy of The Editor, Geriatric Medicine, Modern Medicine GB Ltd

ISBN-13:978-3-540-17056-3 e-ISBN-13:978-1-4471-1432-1
DOI: 10.1007/978-1-4471-1432-1

Phototypesetting by Tradeset Photosetting, 10 Garden Court Business Centre, Tewin Road, Welwyn Garden City, Hertfordshire, AL7 1BH. Printed by Page Bros. (Norwich) Limited, Mile Cross Lane, Norwich.

2128/3916-543210

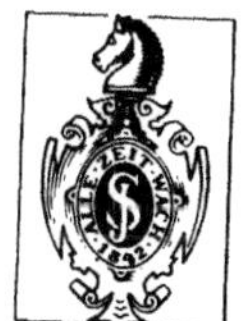

Dedication

To PBG and to my teachers Drs Dunlop, Rodin and Oriel
(DG)

To John and Edna
(SEB)

Preface

"Conclusions are usually considered guesses"
Henry S. Haskins, American writer in *Meditations in Wall Street*

Students' minds, whether undergraduate or postgraduate, soon become stale when faced with lectures or even not so large textbooks. Supplementing lecture notes and textbooks with multiple-choice questions, therefore, attunes the mind to this style of examination which the student will certainly meet and yet also relieves the tedium and monotony of the conventional learning route. This multiple-choice textbook, therefore, should be used side by side with lecture notes, textbooks and clinical teaching material.

The book covers a wide field of genitourinary medicine. This necessarily overlaps with general medicine, urology, bacteriology, virology, psychiatry, sexual medicine, immunology and proctology. With regard to immunology, a basic set of teaching questions are included so that HIV disease may be more easily understood without recourse to immunology textbooks.

The answers to the questions are not given in a uniform style. This is partly to relieve monotony, and partly because some questions need no explanation, others need a prose answer and yet others are best answered by a point-by-point explanation. We also provide references for those interested.

There is some overlap between questions but only enough, we hope, to facilitate learning but not produce somnolence. For the same reason, we have included a sprinkling of cartoons and poems. They all appear in close proximity to the relevant questions in the text. The poems at least are far from works of art, but are designed to make the student think about the pertinent subjects in a lighthearted way and so reinforce the learning process.

The answers to some questions are really clinical opinions, e.g. how to handle frequently recurrent genital herpes. Those who disagree with these or any other answers are invited to write to the authors so that we can be persuaded by their viewpoints.

The Questions and Answers contained in this book have been compiled in collaboration with Drs M. Byrne, G. Forster, S. Forster, D. Hawkins, C. Ison, J. Parkin, L. Stacey, R. Taylor, and Miss A. McCreaner. We should therefore, like to thank all of them for the thought, time and effort they invested in this project.

Grateful thanks are due also to Dr J. R. W. Harris and Dr. A. J. Pinching for their useful comments, to Ann Persad for her typing and to our medical students who have tried out our questions.

London
June 1986

David Goldmeier
Simon Barton

Contents

1. Bacterial Vaginosis, Candidiasis and Trichomoniasis 2
2. Chancroid and Granuloma Inguinale 14
3. Chlamydial Disease 20
4. Colposcopy and Cervical Pathology 30
5. Genital Warts 38
6. Gonorrhoea 44
7. Gastrointestinal Diseases 56
8. Hepatitis 68
9. Genital Herpes 74
10. Human Immunodeficiency Virus (HIV) Related Disease and Immunology 84
11. Pelvic Inflammatory Disease 110
12. Prostatitis 116
13. Psychological and Sexual Problems 122
14. Syphilis 128
15. Miscellaneous 148
16. Case Histories 164

References 184

1. *Bacterial Vaginosis, Candidiasis and Trichomoniasis*

Q.1.1 Bacterial vaginosis is associated with increased numbers of:

a. *Gardnerella vaginalis*
b. Lactobacilli
c. *Mycoplasma hominis*
d. Beta-haemolytic streptococci
e. Non-sporing anaerobes

Q.1.2 'Clue' cells:

a. Are epithelial cells
b. Were described by Gardner and Dukes in 1959
c. Are associated with bacterial vaginosis
d. Are not present in normal women
e. Are covered with lactobacilli

Q.1.3 *Gardnerella vaginalis*:

a. Requires carbon dioxide for growth
b. Produces diffuse beta haemolysis on human blood agar
c. Is always Gram-positive
d. Is only found in women
e. Has been implicated in postpartum endometritis

For answers see over

Answers

A.1.1 a. T
b. F
c. T
d. F
e. T

Bacterial vaginosis is associated with a lack of lactobacilli but an increase in *Gardnerella vaginalis, Mycoplasma hominis* and non-sporing anaerobes. Beta-haemolytic streptococci are not associated with bacterial vaginosis.

A.1.2 a. T
b. T
c. T
d. F
e. F

'Clue' cells which are epithelial cells covered with coccobacilli were first described by Gardner and Dukes in 1959. They are present in large numbers in women with bacterial vaginosis and occur in about 40% of normal women.

A.1.3 a. T
b. T
c. F
d. F
e. T

Gardnerella vaginalis is a Gram-variable bacillus which produces diffuse beta haemolysis on human but not horse blood agar. It has been implicated as the causative agent of bacterial vaginosis and postpartum infection. It is carried in the urethra of 10% of men.

Q.1.4 Bacterial vaginosis:

a. Can be concomitant with trichomonal vaginitis
b. Is treated with erythromycin
c. Is treated with metronidazole
d. Is always symptomatic
e. Is a proven sexually transmitted disease

Q.1.5 Bacterial vaginosis can be diagnosed clinically by the presence of:

a. Vaginal pH 5.0
b. 'Fishy' smell of the vaginal discharge
c. Presence of 'clue' cells
d. Yellow purulent discharge
e. Presence of polymorphs (inflammatory response)

For answers see over

A.1.4 a. T
b. F
c. T
d. F
e. F

Bacterial vaginosis is commonly found in association with trichomonal vaginitis. The treatment of choice is metronidazole; erythromycin is inactive in vivo. Bacterial vaginosis may or may not cause symptoms and has not been proven to be a sexually transmitted infection.

A.1.5 a. T
b. T
c. T
d. F
e. F

Bacterial vaginosis presents clinically with: (1) high pH>4.5, (2) fishy smell of vaginal discharge, (3) large numbers of epithelial cells and 'clue' cells but no polymorphs and (4) white homogeneous discharge.

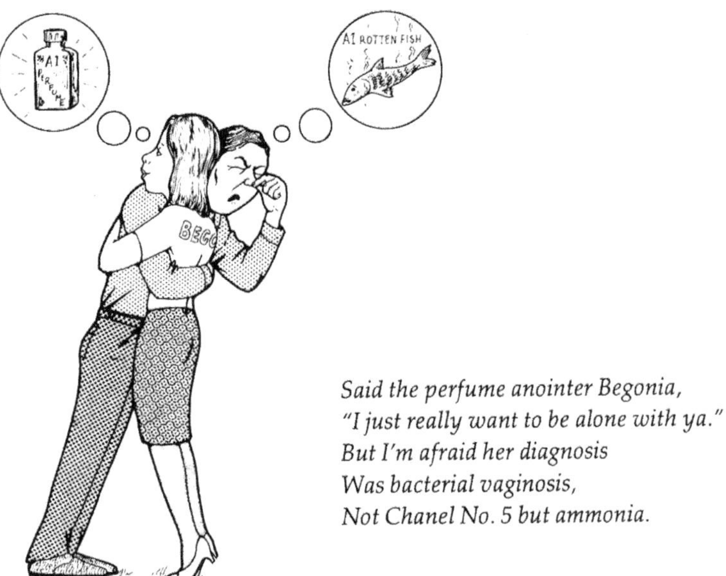

Said the perfume anointer Begonia,
"I just really want to be alone with ya."
But I'm afraid her diagnosis
Was bacterial vaginosis,
Not Chanel No. 5 but ammonia.

Q.1.6 The objective clinical diagnostic criteria for bacterial vaginosis:

a. Are invalid if the patient is menstruating
b. Includes a positive amine test
c. Are dependent on symptoms
d. Include the laboratory culture of *Gardnerella vaginalis* and anaerobic bacteria
e. Include a pH of less than 4.5

Q.1.7 Bacterial vaginosis:

a. Is always sexually transmitted
b. Is strongly associated with the development of pelvic inflammatory disease
c. Is sometimes mistaken clinically for *Trichomonas vaginalis* infection (because of the odour)
d. Occurs in females of all ages
e. Is always associated with the presence of *Gardnerella vaginalis*

Q.1.8 In bacterial vaginosis:

a. A substantial proportion of women are asymptomatic but have objective clinical signs of bacterial vaginosis
b. The vaginal bacteria typically present include *G. vaginalis* and anaerobic bacteria
c. There is a decreased succinate/lactate ratio in vaginal fluid
d. There is an increase in the amines, putrescine and cadaverine present in the vaginal fluid
e. The intrauterine contraceptive device (IUCD) has been implicated as an important risk factor for the development of the condition

For answers see over

A.1.6 a. T
b. T
c. F
d. F
e. F

Three of the four following criteria are required to establish the diagnosis of bacterial vaginosis:

i) A pH value >4.5
ii) A fishy amine odour
iii) The presence of 'clue' cells on microscopy
iv) A low-viscosity homogeneous vaginal discharge

Menstruation may result in both an elevation of pH and production of an amine odour. The presence or absence of various symptoms does not necessarily correlate with the above criteria and a diagnosis based on symptoms confuses the issue.

A.1.7 a. F
b. F
c. T
d. T
e. F

A.1.8 a. T
b. T
c. F
d. T
e. F

There is an increase in the succinate/lactate ratio as measured by gas liquid chromatography. The amines are produced by anaerobic bacteria and cause the malodour.

Q.1.9 The vaginal pH is:

a. Usually between 3.0 and 5.0
b. Raised after sexual intercourse
c. Usually normal in patients with bacterial vaginosis
d. Elevated in postmenopausal women
e. Constant during the menstrual cycle

Q.1.10 The amine test:

a. Is positive in candidiasis
b. Involves adding potassium chloride to the vaginal discharge
c. May be positive during menstruation
d. If positive, is always a sign of infection
e. May be positive in *T. vaginalis* vaginitis

Q.1.11 Which of the following would be likely to result in successful eradication of bacterial vaginosis:

a. Metronidazole 400 mg 12 hourly for 5 days
b. Penicillin V 500 mg 6 hourly for 7 days
c. Povidone iodine pessaries
d. Clotrimazole pessaries
e. Diloxanide furoate 500 mg 8 hourly for 7 days

For answers see over

A.1.9 a. F
b. T
c. F
d. T
e. F

The normal vaginal pH lies within the range of 4.0 and 4.5. Seminal fluid is alkaline and hence sexual intercourse results in a rise in vaginal pH.

pH is raised during and immediately postmenstruation and also in infections with *T. vaginalis* and bacterial vaginosis. The pH also varies with different time of the menstrual cycle, being the highest during menstruation.

A.1.10 a. F
b. F
c. T
d. F
e. T

The amine test involves adding 10% potassium hydroxide solution to the vaginal discharge on a microscope slide, upon which a fishy smell (ammonia) is transiently released.

An amine odour is also found in vaginal fluid in which there is menstrual blood, *T. vaginalis* or semen and hence does not necessarily indicate bacterial vaginosis.

A.1.11 a. T
b. F
c. T
d. F
e. F

The treatment of choice is metronidazole. However, in early pregnancy it is safer to use local povidone iodine which will be likely to result in successful treatment. Penicillin V and clotrimazole are not indicated in bacterial vaginosis. Diloxanide furoate may be used to treat amoebiasis.

Q.1.12 Clinical vaginitis:

a. Is always found in patients colonised with *Candida albicans*
b. Is commonly caused by *Gardnerella vaginalis*
c. May cause dyspareunia
d. Is best treated by a vaginal douche
e. Is often the result of infection with *C. albicans*

Q.1.13 *Candida albicans* in the vagina:

a. Is found in about one-third of normal women
b. May cause dysuria
c. Is characterised by an offensive fishy discharge
d. Raises the vaginal pH above 5
e. Should always be treated

Q.1.14 Infection with *Trichomonas vaginalis* is usually associated with:

a. A reddened vaginal mucosa
b. The likelihood of other concurrent sexually transmitted diseases
c. A thick white non-homogeneous discharge
d. Absence of pus cells on microscopy of vaginal fluid
e. Organisms characteristically seen on Gram-stained preparations of vaginal fluid

For answers see over

A.1.12 a. F
b. F
c. T
d. F
e. T

a. *Candida albicans* colonisation should only be treated if there are symptoms of vaginitis.
b. *Gardnerella vaginalis* interacts with anaerobes to cause a vagin*osis*, not a vagin*itis*.
c. Superficial dyspareunia.
d. False
e. True

A.1.13 a. T
b. T
c. F
d. F
e. F

Vaginitis is usually caused by *C. albicans* or *T. vaginalis* and less commonly by streptococci. It may also result from local chemical irritation.

Candida albicans colonises the vagina of a large proportion of normal women some of whom may be asymptomatic and do not require treatment. The pH is not raised.

A.1.14 a. T
b. T
c. F
d. F
e. F

a. *Trichomonas vaginalis* infection usually causes inflammation.
b. As *T. vaginalis* is a sexually transmitted disease, there is an association between finding it and other STDs.
c. *Trichomonas vaginalis* usually results in a frothy, yellow, offensive and homogeneous discharge, unlike the thick cheesy-white discharge of candidiasis.
d. The presence of an increased number of pus cells on microscopy of the vaginal fluid reflects the inflammatory response to *T. vaginalis*.
e. Mobile trichomonads are seen on examination of the 'wet' film of vaginal fluid seen on either dark-field or light microscopy. They will be missed on a fixed Gram stain.

There once was a virgin from Aberfan,
Who developed some Candida albican(s),
Ampicillin last week,
For infected teeth
Caused curdy discharge and itchan.

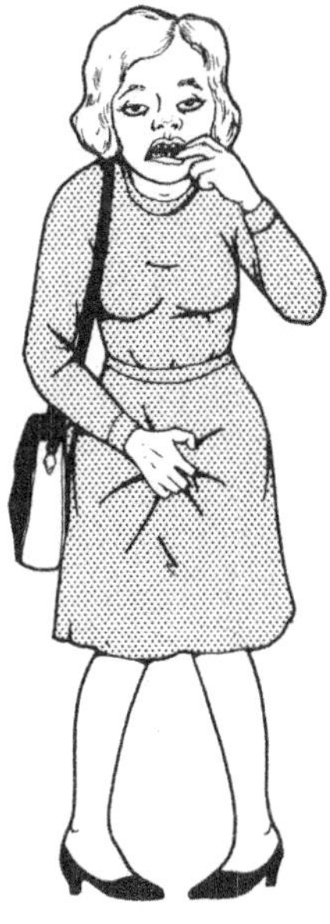

Candida albicans in women causes a white curdy, non-smelly, itchy discharge.

2. *Chancroid and Granuloma Inguinale*

Q.2.1 ***Haemophilus ducreyi*:**

a. Is the causative organism of granuloma inguinale
b. Causes lesions which can lead to autoinoculation
c. Usually appears in chains in a smear taken from a clinical specimen
d. Is said to exacerbate symptoms if coexistent with genital herpes
e. Is a commensal organism

Q.2.2 **The following statements about chancroid are true:**

a. Its highest incidence is in the tropics and subtropics
b. It causes painful deep ulcers with undermined edges
c. If left untreated bubos form in 5% of patients
d. Diagnosis is by culture and/or Giemsa-stained smear of ulcer material
e. Cotrimoxazole, erythromycin and doxycyline may all be effective treatment

Q.2.3 **Granuloma inguinale:**

a. Is caused by *Calymmatobacterium granulomatis*
b. May present as a pruritic nodule on the penis or labia
c. Usually causes local lymphadenopathy
d. May be mistaken for carcinoma of the vulva
e. May remain active for years

For answers see over

Answers

A.2.1
a. F—It is the cause of chancroid.
b. T—Chancroid lesions can autoinoculate on the genital areas or thighs.
c. T
d. T
e. F—It is a pathogen.

A.2.2
a. T
b. T
c. F—It leads to bubo formation in over 60% of patients if left untreated.
d. T
e. T—Treatment failures with tetracyclines and cotrimoxazole have been observed.

A.2.3
a. T
b. T—Early lesions present in this way.
c. F—It never causes lymphadenopathy.
d. T—Ulceration may extend over the vulva, perineum and anal areas, and the edge may be thickened.
e. T

Q.2.4 Management of granuloma inguinale includes:

a. Cleaning the lesions before scraping granulation tissue at its edge to obtain material to make a smear for diagnostic purposes
b. Finding the organism in mononuclear cells in smears
c. Considering it as a diagnostic possibility in travellers from India and Africa
d. Treating the condition with penicillin G i.m.
e. Confirming the diagnosis by means of complement fixation tests on serum

Q.2.5 *Haemophilus ducreyi*:

a. Is the causative organism of chancroid
b. Gives a characteristic Gram stain described as 'shoals of fish'
c. Can successfully be treated with erythromycin
d. Grows well at 37°C
e. Does not carry β-lactamase-coding plasmids

For answers see over

A.2.4 a. T
b. T
c. T
d. F—Tetracyclines and ampicillin may result in successful treatment. However, streptomycin (i.m.) may have to be given in order to achieve a cure. Consider renal function.
e. F—There is no such reliable test.

A.2.5 a. T
b. T
c. T
d. F
e. F

Haemophilus ducreyi classically causes chancroid and is treated with erythromycin. It gives a characteristic Gram stain described as 'shoals of fish', grows at 35°C and can carry β-lactamase-coding plasmids.

3. *Chlamydial Disease*

Q.3.1 Non-gonococcal urethritis (NGU):

a. Like gonococcal urethritis may be asymptomatic
b. Commonly causes microscopic haematuria
c. Is associated with *C. trachomatis* infection in 35%–50% of cases
d. May only be diagnosed, it is generally accepted, when there are at least 15 polymorphonuclear leucocytes (PMNLs) per high-power field (x1000) of Gram-stained urethral smear
e. Is associated with ureaplasma isolation more frequently than with *C. trachomatis* infection in first-attack NGU

Q.3.2 Ophthalmia neonatorum due to *C. trachomatis*

a. Is best treated with systemic tetracyclines
b. Is usually prevented by the prophylactic use of silver nitrate drops (Crede's prophylaxis)
c. Is commonly associated with asymptomatic nasopharyngeal carriage
d. Commonly presents within 3 days of birth
e. Is bilateral in about half of cases

For answers see over

A.3.1 a. T
b. F—Benchside urinalysis should be performed on all first attenders with NGU. If haematuria is present, a midstream urine for bacterial culture should be obtained. An MSU should also be performed if there is increased frequency or nocturia.
c. T
d. F—The generally accepted best cut-off point for significant leucocytosis is now considered to be 5 PMNLs per high-power field (x1000) when the patient has held his urine for 3–4 h.
e. T—About 60% of patients with new attacks of NGU will have ureaplasmas isolated. However, there is evidence that they are not always pathogenic and routine culture for ureaplasmas in NGU is not indicated.

A.3.2 a. F—Systemic tetracyclines are contraindicated in children under 12 years of age due to incorporation of the antibiotic into the dentition. Systemic erythromycin for 2–3 weeks is the preferred treatment as this will successfully eradicate chlamydia both from the eyes and from other sites where there may be asymptomatic carriage (e.g. pharynx). In addition, babies usually present late (3–13 days old) after discharge from hospital and it is difficult for their parents to treat them with eye drops 5–6 times a day for 5–6 weeks.
b. F—Silver nitrate prophylaxis is used to prevent gonococcal ophthalmia (in some parts of the United States).
c. T—See a) above
d. F—See a) above. Gonococcal ophthalmia usually presents within 1–2 days. Early cases of chlamydial ophthalmia have been described in neonates after prolonged rupture of the membranes.
e. T

Q.3.3 The following features favour the diagnosis of acute epididymitis as opposed to torsion of the testis:

a. Tenderness and pain on palpation of a mass posterior to the testis
b. Past history of pain
c. Anterior localisation of epididymis on unaffected side
d. Presence of urethritis and/or pyuria
e. Patient aged 20 years

Chlamydia while doing up her shoe
Was thanked for the very good view.
This caused her to loosen
Her previous twosome
But gave her new friend NSU.

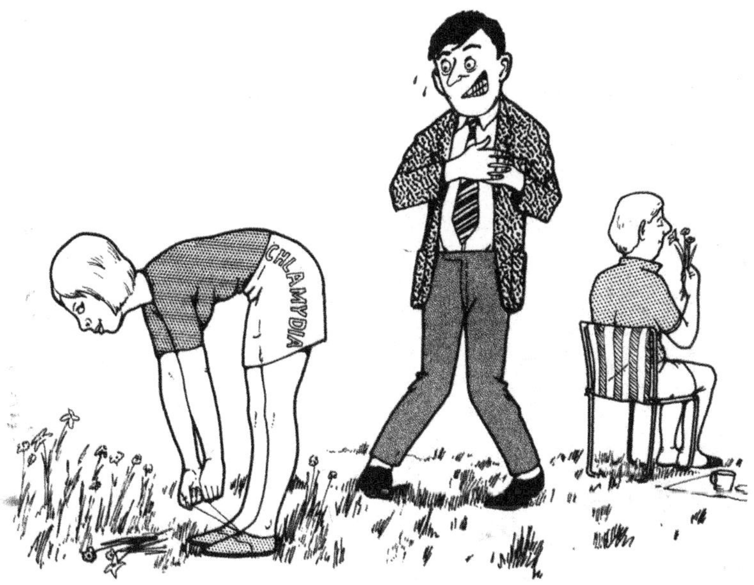

A.3.3 a. T—The epididymis is usually found on the lower and posterior pole of the testis. In epididymitis the testis itself may be relatively spared.

b. F—A past history of pain may suggest episodes of incomplete torsion or past epididymitis which may lead to scarring and chronic mild pain.

c. F—This suggests the possibility of torsion.

d. T

e. F—Could be either. Torsion generally occurs in younger patients.

Q.3.4 Lymphogranulum venereum (LGV):

a. Usually presents with genital ulceration
b. Is caused by certain strains of *Chlamydia psittaci*
c. Responds best to treatment with penicillin
d. Has an incubation period of 3–30 days
e. May be confidently diagnosed if a patient has a positive Frei test

Q.3.5 Sexually acquired reactive arthritis (SARA):

a. Preferentially affects the small joints of the hands
b. Is associated with high chlamydial antibody levels by microimmunofluorescence in more than half of cases
c. Occurs in 1% of patients with NGU
d. Does not occur in women
e. Is commoner in patients with the HLAB-27 histocompatibility antigen

Q.3.6 In lymphogranuloma venereum (LGV):

a. Complement-fixing titres against LGV/psittacosis of greater than 1:64 are found in more than half of the cases
b. Proctitis may occur in both men and women
c. Genital elephantiasis is a recognised complication in the late stages
d. Inguinal bubos occurs more commonly in men than women
e. Inguinal bubos are usually bilateral

For answers see over

A.3.4 a. F—At the lymphadenopathy stage only about 5% of patients have coexisting ulceration and only about one quarter of patients give a history of a genital lesion.
b. F—It is caused by the lymphogranuloma venereum strains of *C. trachomatis* (serovars L1, L2 and L3).
c. F—As with other chlamydial organisms, tetracycline and erythromycin are the antibiotics of choice. Cotrimoxazole has also been used with success. There are little controlled data.
d. T
e. F—The test is based on the intradermal inoculation of heated bubo pus from a case of LGV and is outdated as it is of low sensitivity and specificity.

A.3.5 a. F—The commonest joints affected are the knee, ankle and metatarsophalangeal joints.
b. T—Levels of >1:64 are common and the mean titres for SARA patients as a group are very much higher than in uncomplicated chlamydial NGU, suggesting that chlamydiae are in some way responsible for the reactive arthritis.
c. T
d. F—It occurs rarely in women.
e. T—About 80% of SARA patients have the HLAB-27 antigen.

A.3.6 a. T—Rising titres are rarely seen presumably because the disease is well advanced at clinical presentation.
b. T—In homosexual men severe proctitis may occur early due to direct inoculation of LGV stains. In women proctitis may occur in the late stages of the disease, probably by rectal inoculation from genital infection.
c. T
d. T—Consequently early presentation of the disease occurs much more commonly in men. In women the intra-abdominal nodes may be involved.
e. F

Q.3.7 The conjunctivitis of adult chlamydial ophthalmia (non-trachomatous):

a. Is usually bilateral
b. Cannot be distinguished clinically from adenovirus infection
c. Is totally unresponsive to chloramphenicol eye drops
d. If untreated for greater than 6 months, may lead to blindness
e. Is associated with concurrent chlamydial cervical infection in 90% of women but concurrent urethral infection in only 50% of men

Q.3.8 *Chlamydia trachomatis:*

a. Is an obligate intracellular parasite
b. Organisms are resistant to tetracycline in about 10% of clinical isolates
c. Cervical infection is reliably diagnosed in Papanicolaou (PAP)-stained smears by finding characteristic inclusion bodies
d. May be found in about 25% of men at the time of diagnosis of gonococcal urethritis
e. Is a significant cause of acute prostatitis

Q.3.9 Non-gonococcal urethritis (NGU):

a. Is the same as non-specific urethritis (NSU)
b. Is rarely caused by herpes simplex virus
c. Is rarely caused by a urinary tract infection
d. May be treated with rifampicin or erythromycin
e. Is chronic in 5%–10% of men

For answers see over

A.3.7 a. F—Only about one-third of cases are bilateral.
b. T—Even with slit lamp examination it appears identical (i.e. has "follicle" formation).
c. F—Chloramphenicol has some antichlamydial effect but is inadequate for definitive treatment.
d. F—Despite great similarity between trachoma (A–C) serovars and oculogenital (D–K) serovars additional factors seem to be required other than simple chlamydial infection for progression to pannus formation. Low-grade follicular conjunctivitis may, however, persist for months to years if untreated in the D–K-type infection.
e. T

A.3.8 a. T
b. F—*Chlamydia trachomatis* microorganisms have never been known to be resistant to either tetracycline or erythromycin.
c. F—Inclusion bodies seen on cervical PAP smear are neither sensitive nor specific indicators of chlamydial infection.
d. T—*Chlamydia trachomatis* is a common cause of post-gonococcal urethritis.
e. F—It has rarely been found in prostatic fluid, but it is difficult to say if this is contamination from the urethra or not.

A.3.9 a. F—All male urethritis not due to the gonococcus is NGU, e.g. herpes simplex virus and urinary tract infection. When all causes of male urethritis are excluded (*C. trachomatis* in 40%, herpes simplex virus (<1%), meatal warts (<1%), meatal chancre (<1%), urinary tract infection (<1%)), the urethritis is of unknown aetiology and is then said to be non-specific (NSU).
b. T—See a) above.
c. T—The patient usually complains of increased frequency, urgency and burning micturition as well as having urethritis.
d. F—If rifampicin is given on its own, there is a theoretical risk of resistance developing. This drug should be reserved for anti-TB therapy.
e. T

A Sonnet to Male Urinary Tract Infection
(apologies to WS)

Shall I compare thee to NSU?
Thou urine art more painful and more frequent,
Rough rigors do shake the over 42s,
But for VD the patients seeketh his treatment,
Sometimes too hot the male urethral feels,
And urine's clear complexion clouded be,
Not all urethral discharge from the act sequaels,
But by chance does E. coli *to the bladder flee,*
But thy continuous discharge shall not fade,
Unless from tetracycline tabs thou changest,
But E. coli *brag he wondr'st in the bladdr'y shade*
When in the urethra thou thinks chlamydia growest.

So long as trimethoprim does not the patient see,
So long lives E. coli *and infection in the wee.*

4. *Colposcopy and Cervical Pathology*

Q.4.1 The following infections are associated with development of cervical cancer:

a. Gonorrhoea
b. Genital warts
c. Candidiasis
d. Herpes genitalis
e. Trichomonasis

Q.4.2 The following factors are *not* associated with an increased risk of developing cervical intraepithelial neoplasia:

a. Multiple sexual partners
b. Early age of first intercourse
c. Smoking tobacco
d. Repeated episodes of bacterial vaginosis
e. Oral herpes simplex infection

Q.4.3 Common causes of a clinical cervicitis are:

a. Cytomegalovirus infection
b. Human papilloma virus infection
c. Gonorrhoea
d. *Chlamydia trachomatis*
e. Herpes simplex virus infection

Q.4.4 Annual cervical smears for cytology are recommended for the following groups of women:

a. Prostitutes
b. Women with genital warts
c. Grand multipara
d. Women with recurrent bacterial vaginosis
e. Women whose regular sexual partner has genital warts

For answers see over

Answers

A.4.1 a. F
b. T—Human papilloma virus is thought to be directly oncogenic, most notably type 16.
c. F
d. T—There is an association which is not thought to be directly causative between carcinoma of the cervix and past genital herpes.
e. F

A.4.2 a. F
b. F
c. F
d. T
e. T

A.4.3 a. F
b. F
c. T
d. T
e. T

A.4.4 a. T
b. T
c. F
d. F
e. T

Recent studies suggest that women in the above risk groups should have annual colposcopic examination of their lower genital tract. However, as yet limited resources confine this service to research projects.

Q.4.5 Colposcopy is best performed:

a. On or about day 3 of the menstrual cycle
b. Before taking a routine cervical smear
c. Mid-cycle
d. In conjunction with taking a cervical smear
e. With the aim of obtaining directed biopsies for histological diagnosis

Q.4.6 Cytological examination of a Papanicolaou cervical smear has a high specificity in diagnosing the following:

a. Bacterial vaginosis
b. Gonorrhoea
c. Herpes simplex virus infection
d. Human papilloma virus infection
e. Actinomycosis

Q.4.7 Cervical columnar epithelium:

a. Is five to ten cells thick
b. Does not produce mucus
c. Stains dark brown after application of Lugol's iodine
d. Has a typical "cluster of grapes" appearance
e. Always lines the entire endocervical canal

For answers see over

A.4.5 a. F—Colposcopy should not be performed during menstruation.
b. F—Colposcopy is not designed to replace cytological screening. It should be performed following the report of a suspicious smear.
c. T—This is the ideal time to perform colposcopy, as the external os is wide open.
d. F—As stated above, colposcopy is an additional method available to study cervical disease. Smear results should be available prior to the examination.
e. T—In addition to identifying the extent of the abnormal epithelium, this is the main aim of the colposcopist.

A.4.6 a. F
b. F
c. T—large multinucleate giant cells reliably diagnose HSV infections.
d. T—Koilocytes (vacuolated epithelial cells) are indicative of wart virus (HPV) infection.
e. F

a), b) and e) cannot reliably be diagnosed on a Papanicolaou smear.

c) and d) do not have a high sensitivity, but are highly specific for their respective infections if found.

A.4.7 a. F—It is one cell thick. Squamous epithelium is 15–20 cells thick.
b. F—Columnar epithelium produces mucus.
c. F—Columnar epithelium does not take up the iodine stain as it does not contain glycogen.
d. T—The glandular mucosa is not smooth. It covers numerous connective tissue papillae, thus giving an appearance of numerous minute polyps.
e. F—The squamocolumnar junction can lie in the cervical canal, and therefore some squamous epithelium can line the lower end of the canal. This occurs after the menopause or following local destructive therapy (e.g. cone biopsy or diathermy).

Q.4.8 The squamocolumnar junction (SCJ) of the cervix:

a. Is always visible at colposcopy
b. Is a junction between a 16-cell-thick and a 1-cell-thick epithelium
c. Becomes more ectocervical after the menopause
d. Becomes endocervical with the use of oestrogens
e. Is the only site of Nabothian follicles

Q.4.9 The following are features of an atypical transformation zone on the cervix:

a. Whitening after application of acetic acid
b. Lack of mosaic pattern
c. Punctuation pattern
d. Nabothian follicles
e. Complete uptake of Lugol's iodine

For answers see over

A.4.8 a. F—The site of the SCJ is variable, and therefore not always visible if situated within the endocervical canal.
b. T
c. F—After the menopause, due to lack of oestrogens, the cervix atrophies and involutes. Thus the SCJ recedes up the canal.
d. F—The SCJ becomes more ectocervical (also at puberty and during pregnancy).
e. F—Nabothian follicles arise in the columnar epithelium and are therefore also found in the transformation zone, not just along the SCJ.

A.4.9 a. T—This is the typical reaction of abnormal epithelium.
b. F—Lack of mosaic pattern is the appearance of a *typical* transformation zone.
c. T—Both the mosaic and punctuation patterns represent the abnormal vascular patterns.
d. F—These are features of a normal transformation zone.
e. F—The reverse is true. Abnormal squamous epithelium does not contain glycogen, and therefore fails to take up the stain.

5. *Genital Warts*

Q.5.1 Widespread vaginal warts can be safely and effectively treated with:

a. Liquid nitrogen
b. Laser therapy
c. Twenty-five per cent podophyllin applied topically
d. Cryosurgery
e. Systemic acyclovir

Q.5.2 Genital warts usually:

a. Are unilateral
b. Regress spontaneously within a month
c. Are transmitted by sexual contact
d. Are decreasing in incidence in the UK
e. Will increase in size during pregnancy

Q.5.3 Human papilloma virus (HPV) is responsible for:

a. Condylomata lata
b. White patches on the cervix
c. Polyps on the cervix
d. Koilocytes on cervical smears
e. Cervical ectropion

Q.5.4 Vulval warts:

a. Have an incubation period of up to 90 days
b. Are associated with marked vaginal discharge
c. Cause inguinal lymphadenopathy
d. Are infectious to a sexual partner
e. Are not associated with abnormal cervical smears

For answers see over

Answers

A.5.1
a. T
b. T
c. F—This is not recommended because there may be a significant absorption of podophyllin where it is used over a wide area. This may lead to neurotoxicity.
d. T
e. F—There is no evidence that acyclovir acts on the human papilloma virus.

A.5.2
a. F—They can occur anywhere in the anogenital area.
b. F—It is unusual for genital warts to resolve within a month.
c. T—Self-inoculation can occur (e.g. from warts on the hand), but genital warts are usually acquired at sexual intercourse.
d. F—There is an increase in incidence in the UK, but this increase also reflects an increased awareness of the condition among patients and doctors.
e. T—But they usually resolve quickly and spontaneously after pregnancy.

A.5.3
a. F—HPV is responsible for condylomata acuminata. Condylomata lata are caused by secondary syphilis.
b. T—HPV can commonly cause flat warts on the cervix which are seen as white patches.
c. F—HPV can also cause condylomatous lesions on the cervix. Polyps are tumours of mucous membrane NOT caused by HPV.
d. T—Koilocytes are diagnostic of HPV infection.
e. F—Cervical ectropion is caused by the presence of columnar epithelium on the ectocervix.

A.5.4
a. T
b. F—Vulval warts do not cause a marked vaginal discharge.
c. F
d. T
e. F—Fifty per cent of patients with vulval warts have abnormal exfoliative cervical cytology.

Q.5.5 Twenty-five per cent podophyllin (dissolved in methanol), a local cytotoxic agent:

a. Can usually be used to treat keratotic vulval warts
b. Should be kept on vulval warts for 12 h before washing off at the initial application
c. Can safely be used to treat vulval warts in pregnant women
d. May be kept on vulval warts for up to 24 h in resistant cases
e. May be neurotoxic

Q.5.6 DNA hybridisation techniques have:

a. Shown human papilloma virus (HPV) types 6 and 11 to be associated with wart virus infection of the cervix
b. Shown HPV 16 and 18 to be associated with carcinoma of the cervix
c. Enabled HPV to be grown in the laboratory
d. Been carried out in situ, i.e. in tissue sections
e. Enabled HPV to be found in juvenile laryngeal papillomas

Q.5.7 In the treatment of anogenital warts:

a. Podophyllin 25% should be used to treat cervical warts
b. Podophyllin should be washed off any time up to 24 h later
c. An excess of podophyllin may be very cardiotoxic
d. Anal warts may be cut off with scissors
e. Anal warts are often the easiest to treat of all warts

For answers see over

A.5.5 a. F—Where genital warts are keratotic, there is usually little or no clinical response to local podophyllin.
b. F—Because of some patient's marked sensitivity to podophyllin, it should be left in situ for no more than 3 h on the first application.
c. F—There are reports of neurotoxicity and stillbirth following its use in pregnancy.
d. T—Where there is a clinical response and no sensitivity, podophyllin may be left in situ for up to 24 h. If soreness occurs, this may be controlled by application of local weak steroid creams for a few days after washing off the podophyllin.
e. T—In large amounts it may be neurotoxic.

A.5.6 a. T
b. T
c. F—HPV cannot be grown in vitro. This is one of the reasons why the hybridisation technique was developed for this virus, i.e. to classify it according to clinical findings and DNA analysis.
d. T
e. T

A.5.7 a. F—Cervical warts should not be treated with podophyllin because of the theoretical risk of oncogenicity.
b. T—Podophyllin should be washed off any time up to 24 h after application. A test dose should be given and washed off 3 h later.
c. F—Podophyllin is very neurotoxic in large local amounts.
d. T—The "scissor technique" is to infiltrate the anal area with weak adrenaline, causing the warts to be proud of the skin and then cut them off with scissors.
e. F—Anal warts are the most difficult to treat of all warts.

WARTS
HPV16

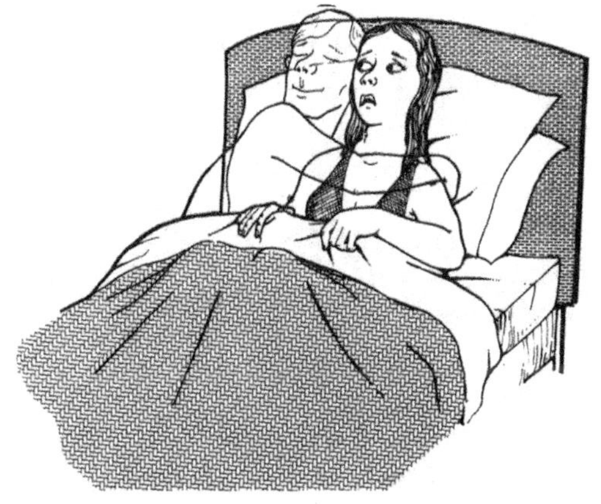

While sleeping alone late one night,
Linda dreamt of a sexual fright
That her Joe had a wart,
Indeed one that he'd caught,
And if type 16 would not *be alright.*

6. *Gonorrhoea*

Q.6.1 Selective agents used in culture media for the isolation of *Neisseria gonorrhoeae* include:

a. Lincomycin
b. Penicillin
c. Cephalosporins
d. Trimethroprim
e. Nystatin

Q.6.2 The 2.6-Md (megadalton) plasmid found in *N. gonorrhoeae*:

a. Has no known function
b. Mediates conjugation
c. Carries the code for β-lactamase
d. Is present in at least 90% of strains
e. Is unstable

Q.6.3 Strains of *N. gonorrhoeae* that cause disseminated gonococcal infection (DGI) typically:

a. Are resistant to penicillin
b. Are resistant to killing by normal human serum
c. Require arginine, hypoxanthine and uracil for growth
d. Form transparent colony phenotypes
e. Are isolated from blood cultures in >80% of cases

For answers see over

A.6.1 a. T
b. F
c. F
d. T
e. T

Lincomycin suppresses Gram-positive organisms, trimethoprim Gram-negative organisms (but only occasionally *N. gonorrhoeae*) and nystatin inhibits *Candida* sp. Penicillin would inhibit both normal flora and gonococci.

A.6.2 a. T
b. F
c. F
d. T
e. F

The 2.6-Md plasmid is found in >90% of *N. gonorrhoeae* and has no known function.

A.6.3 a. F
b. T
c. T
d. T
e. F—*Neissaria gonorrhoeae* is isolated in blood from considerably less than 80% of cases of DGI.

Strains of *N. gonorrhoeae* that cause DGI have particular characteristics:

1) Are highly susceptible to penicillin
2) Are resistant to killing by normal human serum
3) Require arginine, hypoxanthine and uracil for growth
4) Form transparent colony types

Q.6.4 Disseminated gonococcal infection:

a. Is more common in men
b. Only results from repeated infection
c. Can occur in patients with deficiency of one of the late-acting complement components
d. Can present as septic arthritis
e. Is not affected by hormonal influences

Q.6.5 Beta-lactamase (penicillinase) production in *N. gonorrhoeae*:

a. Is due to a chromosomal mutation
b. Is plasmid mediated
c. Gives high levels of penicillin resistance
d. Resistance is not affected by the inoculum used for testing
e. Can be detected using a chromogenic cephalosporin

Q.6.6 Penicillinase-producing *N. gonorrhoeae* (PPNG) infections:

a. Originated in the Far East and Africa
b. Should be treated with high doses of ampicillin
c. Do not cause DGI
d. Are more prevalent in homosexuals
e. Are sensitive to treatment with cephalosporins

For answers see over

A.6.4 a. F
b. F
c. T
d. T
e. F

Disseminated gonococcal infection is more common in women who present at the time of onset of menstruation. Patients with a complement deficiency are particularly susceptible.

A.6.5 a. F
b. T
c. T
d. F
e. T

Penicillinase production in *N. gonorrhoeae* is plasmid mediated. It gives high levels of resistance which varies with the bacterial concentration (i.e. inoculum). A chromogenic cephalosporin (nitrocefin test) is used in the laboratory for rapid identification of penicillinase — the reagent turns from yellow to pink for positive. The commonest cause of penicillin resistance in *N. gonorrhoeae* in the UK at present is chromosomally directed — not plasmid (penicillinase producer) controlled.

A.6.6 a. T
b. F
c. F
d. F
e. T

Penicillinase-producing *N. gonorrhoeae* originated as separate but simultaneous events in the Far East and Africa. They are rarely isolated from homosexuals and are treated with either spectinomycin or a cephalosporin.

Q.6.7 ***Neisseria gonorrhoeae* require for growth:**

a. Five to 7% carbon dioxide
b. Anaerobic atmosphere
c. Low humidity
d. Source of iron
e. Temperature of 36°C

Q.6.8 ***Neisseria gonorrhoeae* can be typed for epidemiological purposes by:**

a. Nutritional requirements
b. Utilisation of carbohydrates
c. Using monoclonal antibodies
d. Outer membrane protein I
e. Enzyme profiles

John the medic's great fear
Was getting resistant gonorrhoea,
The plasmids demise
And chromosomal surprise
Meant girls out so he poured forth the beer.

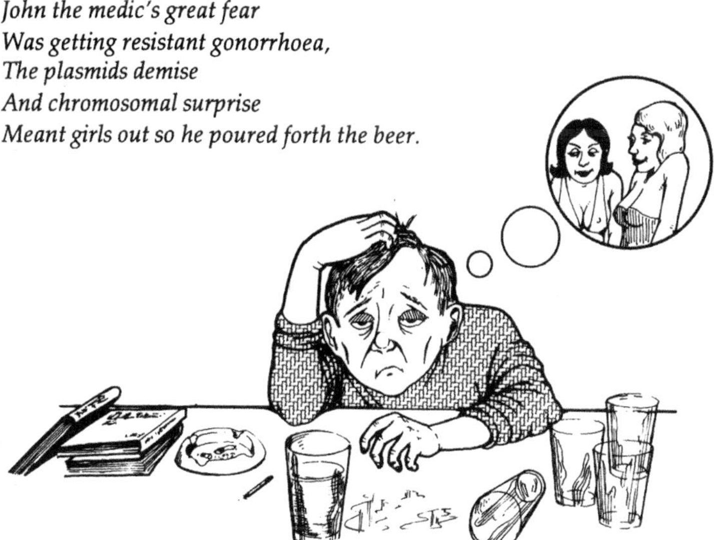

A.6.7 a. T
b. F
c. F
d. T
e. T

Neisseria gonorrhoeae require 5%–7% carbon dioxide, high humidity, a temperature of 36°–37°C and a source of iron for growth.

A.6.8 a. T
b. F
c. T
d. T
e. F

Neisseria gonorrhoeae can be typed by:

1) Nutritional requirements (auxotyping)
2) Monoclonal antibodies raised to two epitopes on the outer membrane protein 1

Q.6.9 The use of the Gram stain in the diagnosis of gonorrhoea:

a. Is positive when *only* intracellular diplococci are seen
b. Is regarded positive if *any* diplococci are seen
c. Is particularly useful in rectal gonorrhoea
d. In male urethral samples has a sensitivity of 90%
e. In female cervical samples has a sensitivity of 80%

Q.6.10 Gonococcal pharyngitis:

a. Can only occur after fellatio
b. Is often asymptomatic
c. Cannot be diagnosed on a Gram-stain smear of pharyngeal exudate
d. Rarely resolves spontaneously
e. Is often resistant to conventional treatment for gonorrhoea
f. Never leads to gonococcal dissemination

Q.6.11 The following is true about gonorrhoea:

a. It may be diagnosed on the basis of a Gram-stained smear of urethral exudate in about 89% of men
b. It may be diagnosed on the basis of a Gram-stained smear of urethral exudate in about 35% of men
c. It may be diagnosed on the basis of a Gram-stained smear of urethral and/or cervical material in up to 60% of women
d. It may be diagnosed on the basis of a Gram-stained smear of urethral and/or cervical material in up to 35% of women
e. Direct monoclonal antibody staining of cervical material is less sensitive than Gram-stained preparations

For answers see over

A.6.9 a. T
b. F
c. F
d. T
e. F

The Gram stain is indicative of gonorrhoea if Gram-negative intracellular diplococci are seen. It has a sensitivity of >90% in symptomatic males and 40%–50% in asymptomatic males, females and rectal gonorrhoea.

A.6.10 a. F—*Neisseria gonorrhoeae* infection of the tonsils and pharynx is usually acquired at fellatio but less commonly by cunnilingus.
b. T—It is often asymptomatic but may present as acute tonsilitis with exudate, cervical lymphadenopathy, pharyngeal pain or fever.
c. T—A Gram-stained smear of pharyngeal material may reveal Gram-negative intracellular diplococci but this may be caused by other, often commensal neisserial infection (e.g. *N. lactamicus*); thus culture or other confirmatory techniques are needed to make the diagnosis.
d. F—Gonococcal pharyngitis usually resolves without treatment within a few weeks.
e. T—Pharyngeal infection responds relatively poorly to spectinomycin and ampicillin plus probenecid.
f. F—It may rarely lead to disseminated gonococcal infection, e.g. septic arthritis.

A.6.11 a. T
b. F
c. T
d. F
e. F—Monoclonal antibody stains of direct smears are more sensitive than Gram-stain preparations in females (in males of equal sensitivity).

Q.6.12 Gonococcal urethritis in men:

a. Is usually asymptomatic
b. Causes a yellow purulent urethral discharge
c. Has an incubation period of about 3 days
d. May cause a secondary balanitis
e. May be homosexually acquired by anal intercourse or fellatio

Q.6.13 The site most likely to yield gonococci in women is:

a. The cervix
b. The urethra
c. The rectum
d. The pharynx
e. Posterior vaginal fornix

Q.6.14 Disseminated gonococcal infection:

a. May present with a rash on the extremities over the joints which may appear as small pustular or haemorrhagic lesions
b. May cause an intermittent fever
c. May lead to purulent arthritis
d. May lead to purulent pharyngitis
e. Causes profound thrombocytopenia

For answers see over

A.6.12 a. F
b. T
c. T
d. T
e. T

A.6.13 a. T
b. F
c. F
d. F
e. F

A.6.14 a. T
b. T
c. T
d. F
e. F

7. *Gastrointestinal Diseases*

Q.7.1 In the AIDS-related complex, which of the following are true about the oral cavity or fundus oculi:

a. "Thrush" (oral candida) is common
b. Retinal exudates may affect vision
c. Kaposi's sarcoma may present initially in the mouth
d. Wart-like lesions, hairy oral leukoplakia (HAL), are found on the anterior aspect of the tongue
e. HIV may be found in saliva

Q.7.2 Large-volume watery diarrhoea without blood or mucus in patients with AIDS or the AIDS-related complex (ARC) is likely to be due to:

a. Cytomegalovirus
b. *Shigella* spp.
c. *Campylobacter* spp.
d. Is of unknown aetiology
e. Has been associated with finding candida in small bowel biopsies

Q.7.3 The following points about *Giardia lamblia* are true:

a. It causes a proctitis
b. It is a cause of intestinal malabsorption
c. It may be acquired sexually
d. It may be found in the water supplies in some of the world's cities
e. It may be treated with broad-spectrum antibiotics

Q.7.4 Cryptosporidium is a parasite that:

a. Often causes profuse watery diarrhoea
b. Is commonly a fatal illness in homosexual men with AIDS
c. Is relatively easy to treat
d. Is treated with metronidazole
e. Never causes illness in the non-immunocompromised

For answers see over

Answers

A.7.1 a. T—White adherent plaque may be seen on the lateral side and underneath the tongue in early cases, and throughout the oral cavity in late cases.
b. T—Retinal exudates, often due to cytomegalovirus, but sometimes of unknown aetiology, are commonly found in the macular area.
c. T—Commonly on the hard or soft palate.
d. F—These lesions (HAL) are found on the lateral border of the tongue and are thought to be due to EB virus.
e. T

A.7.2 a. F—a), b), and c) all cause a proctocolitis (blood and mucus).
b. F—See a) above.
c. F—See a) above.
d. T—To date the diarrhoea is of unknown aetiology.
e. T

A.7.3 a. F—*Giardia lamblia* infests the upper small gut.
b. T—It is a cause of malabsorption.
c. T—Oroanal intercourse, particularly between homosexuals, is a mode of transfer.
d. T—Many of the world's cities, particularly outside North America and Europe, have these pathogens in the water supply.
e. F—It may be eradicated by giving metronidazole orally 2.0 g/day for 3 days.

A.7.4 a. T—The coccidian parasite cryptosporidium causes profuse watery diarrhoea.
b. T—It is a fatal illness in homosexual men with AIDS.
c. F—There is no known effective treatment although spiramycin was thought to be useful at one stage.
d. F—See c) above
e. F—It is known to affect immunocompetent patients, causing a self-limiting diarrhoeal illness. The incidence of it in diarrhoeal illnesses is unknown.

Q.7.5 The following organisms are generally accepted as causing proctocolitis in homosexual men:

a. *Campylobacter* spp.
b. Streptococci
c. *Shigella* spp.
d. *Chlamydia trachomatis*
e. *Entamoeba coli*

Q.7.6 *Chlamydia proctitis*:

a. May be clinically silent
b. May be diagnosed by monoclonal antibody stain
c. Is seen in women and homosexual men
d. Always needs treatment
e. Is thought to be the cause for the recent increase in anal carcinomas in homosexual men

Q.7.7 Gonococcal proctitis in homosexual men:

a. Is acquired transintestinally from orogenital intercourse
b. Usually causes malaise
c. Is as easily diagnosed on a Gram stain of rectal exudate as male gonococcal urethral exudate
d. Should be treated by a loading dose of antibiotic
e. If caused by a penicillinase-producing organism, should be treated with flucloxacillin

For answers see over

A.7.5 a. T—*Campylobacter* spp. cause proctocolitis.
b. F—Not known specifically to infect the rectum or colon.
c. T—*Shigella* spp. cause proctocolitis.
d. T—*Chlamydia trachomatis* serovar D–K generally causes proctitis only. Types LGV I, II, III also infect the descending colon and rectum.
e. F—*Entamoeba coli* is a non-pathogenic protozoan.

A.7.6 a. T—*Chlamydia proctitis,* when caused by an LGV strain, usually causes severe proctitis with accompanying symptoms. Proctitis due to D–K serotype may be clinically silent, with the mucosa showing no inflammatory change to the naked eye and histologically.
b. T—Certain cell surface antigens of *C. trachomatis* provide a specific site of attachment for monoclonal antibodies which may be used diagnostically on a smear of rectal exudate. Its sensitivity and specificity remain to be evaluated in that site.
c. T—Both homosexual men and women can develop chlamydial proctitis.
d. T—If left untreated it may produce severe proctitis and may be a source of infection to others.
e. F—*Chlamydia trachomatis* causes a proctitis. The supposed recent increase in *anal* carcinomas is, therefore, not due to this agent.

A.7.7 a. F—Gonococcal proctitis results from introduction of *Neisseria gonorrhoeae* into the rectum directly at intercourse.
b. F—Is usually asymptomatic.
c. F—The sensitivity of a Gram-stained specimen of urethral gonorrhoea is about 90% in men. That of rectal gonorrhoea is at best about 50%.
d. T—Treatment of rectal gonorrhoea is best done with a loading dose of antibiotic to obviate the need for strict patient compliance. Beta-lactamase gonococci responds to spectinomycin and penicillin-sensitive organisms to a loading dose of ampicillin and probenecid.
e. F—Flucloxacillin is not an appropriate antibiotic for treating β-lactamase gonorrhoea.

Q.7.8 In the United States and the United Kingdom *Entamoeba histolytica* excretion:

a. Has a prevalence of 10% of the total population
b. Is as likely to reflect foreign travel in a heterosexual as it is to reflect oroanal intercourse in a homosexual man
c. Is more likely to be confirmed if three stools rather than one are examined
d. Is a recognised cause of protein malabsorption
e. May be clinically indistinguishable from idiopathic ulcerative colitis

Q.7.9 *Giardia lamblia* is:

a. Usually unaffected by gastric acid
b. Not uncommonly causes an asymptomatic infection
c. Treated with metronidazole
d. Not uncommonly coexists with *E. histolytica* in homosexual men
e. A common cause of colitis

Q.7.10 Severe symptomatic infectious proctitis (without colitis) in homosexual men usually causes:

a. Tenesmus
b. Loose water stools
c. Mucosal appearance clinically indistinguishable from ulcerative proctitis
d. Bloody rectal mucosal discharge
e. Faecal constipation

For answers see over

A.7.8 a. F—In the United States and the United Kingdom *E. histolytica* is found in the faeces of less than 1% of the whole population.

b. T—Work from New York in the 1970s showed that excretors were either male homosexuals who had not been abroad or heterosexuals who had travelled to other parts of the world where *E. histolytica* is endemic (e.g. Mexico, S. Africa, India).

c. T—The cornerstone of diagnosis is competent stool examination for parasite. This is most effectively done on several fresh purged stool specimens at 2–3 day intervals.

d. F—*Entamoeba histolytica* does not cause small bowel disease.

e. T—In severe cases of amoebic colitis the mucosa may be diffusely haemorrhagic and ulcerated, resembling ulcerative colitis.

A.7.9 a. F—Gastric acid actually appears to facilitate excystation.

b. T—In adults *G. lamblia* frequently produces very few symptoms. However, it may result in an increase in bulk of faeces or only excessive flatus and cramps.

c. T—Metronidazole (2.0 g a day for 3 days) usually results in elimination of this pathogen.

d. T—About a third of homosexual men attending VD clinics in New York excreted *G. lamblia, E. histolytica* or both.

e. F—*Giardia lamblia* affects the small bowel particularly the jejunum not colon.

A.7.10 a. T—Symptomatic severe proctitis means inflammation of the rectum not usually higher than the sigmoid junction. Severe proctitis causes rectal pain, rectal discharge (blood and/or mucus), constipation and tenesmus (an intense urge to defaecate with little or no result).

b. F—Severe proctitis renders the rectum almost functionless, so that there is faecal constipation.

c. T—A red, oedematous appearance is usually found in the rectum of patients with severe infectious proctitis and ulcerative colitis.

d. T—See a) above

e. T—See a) above

Q.7.11 Gonococcal proctitis:

a. Is usually symptomatic
b. May arise from gonococcal cervicitis via secretions contaminating the perineum and anus
c. Rarely if ever involves the descending colon
d. Is the only site positive in women in 50% of cases
e. Is likely to be successfully treated with tetracycline

Q.7.12 The following are true of *E. histolytica*:

a. It is a cause of proctocolitis and liver abscesses
b. Different biotypes of this protozoan exist
c. Just over 30% of homosexual men in the United States and the United Kingdom excrete it in faeces
d. Is more likely to be identified in trophozoite form in solid faeces than in liquid
e. May be treated with metronidazole

For answers see over

A.7.11 a. F—There is a spectrum of rectal inflammatory response to *N. gonorrhoeae,* ranging from severe proctitis (symptomatic) to no inflammation at all. However, gonococcal proctitis is usually asymptomatic.

b. T—Contamination of the everted anus by cervical secretions during defaecation has been proposed as the general and common mechanism for autoinoculation but rectal intercourse in women who attend clinics may not be uncommon.

c. T—The gonococcus never invades higher than the lower few centimetres of the rectum, unless trauma, e.g. fisting, has caused infection higher up.

d. F—It is the only site positive in about 5% of women.

e. F—β-lactamase gonococci are not commonly found in the rectum. Sensitive strains in homosexual men almost always respond to spectinomycin 2.0 g or ampicillin 3.5 g with probenecid (5% failure rate). Tetracycline may result in a failure rate as high as 30%.

A.7.12 a. T—This occurs particularly in Africa, India and South America.

b. T—Enzyme types — zymodemes — are the method of classification. Some zymodemes appear to be "pathogenic", others "non-pathogenic".

c. F—About 10% of homosexual men excrete EH in faeces

d. F—Trophozoites are very unlikely to be found in solid faeces so that isolation rates increase if the faeces are purged.

e. T—Up to 800 mg 8 hourly for 10 days is needed for eradication of EH.

Q.7.13 The following statements about rigid sigmoidoscopy in relation to STDs are true:

a. It gives a clear view of the whole of the rectum up to the rectosigmoid junction
b. Biopsy through the sigmoidscope is safer on the posterior rather than the anterior rectal wall
c. Early syphilis of the rectum has characteristic histological changes of endarteritis and chronic inflammatory cell infiltrate
d. Postrectal biopsy aerosol blood spray from flatus passing over the lesion may be dangerous to the operator because of potential HIV infection
e. Rectal Kaposi's sarcoma (KS) and CMV proctitis both may be diagnosed on rectal biopsy histopathology and both may respond to treatment

For answers see over

A.7.13 a. F—From distal to proximal the anorectal canal travels anteriorly then posteriorly and upwards to follow the sacral curve. Therefore, the posterior rectal wall just above the anorectal junction may not be visible at sigmoidoscopy.

b. T—The peritoneal reflection comes lower down on the anterior than posterior rectal wall; hence the risk of perforation and peritonitis at biopsy is greater at anterior wall biopsy.

c. T

d. T—The risk of acquiring HIV-related disease by bloody aerosol spray at endoscopy is small but very real. A mask and goggles should be worn for this procedure.

e. F—Kaposi's sarcoma and CMV both need deep biopsies and both are at least to some extent treatable manifestations of AIDS (KS with alpha interferon, CMV with DHPG, a new anti-CMV drug).

8. *Hepatitis*

Q.8.1 Hepatitis B:

a. Has an incubation period of 6 weeks to 3 months in the majority of cases
b. Is always associated with jaundice
c. Is usually transmitted by contamination of food
d. Confers immunity on those infected in the majority of cases
e. May be prevented by immunisation

Q.8.2 In acute viral hepatitis:

a. Fever is common in hepatitis B
b. Arthralgia, usually affecting several small joints, occurs in 25% of patients with hepatitis B
c. Rashes are present in 10% of patients with acute hepatitis
d. The spleen is palpable in 10%–15% of patients with acute hepatitis
e. Epstein–Barr virus infection is a cause of non-A, non-B hepatitis

Q.8.3 Following acute viral hepatitis:

a. Relapses of acute infection of hepatitis are more common following hepatitis B than other types
b. Chronic liver disease is a complication of hepatitis A
c. Women are more likely to become carriers of hepatitis B than men
d. Five to 10% of adults become carriers of hepatitis B
e. Life-long immunity develops after both hepatitis A and hepatitis B in immunocompetent patients

Q.8.4 Hepatitis B may be transmitted by:

a. The use of shared unsterile needles and syringes
b. The faecal-oral route
c. The sharing of a razor with an infected individual
d. The vertical route from mother to infant
e. The sexual route

For answers see over

Answers

A.8.1
a. T
b. F—Patients with chronic hepatitis B are anicteric.
c. F—Hepatitis A may be transmitted by this route. Hepatitis B is transmitted via blood or blood products and sexually, particularly between male homosexuals.
d. T
e. T—Both active and passive vaccines are available.

A.8.2
a. F—Fever up to 38.5°C is common in hepatitis A.
b. T
c. T—Rashes described as erythematous, macular or maculopapular occur in 10% of cases of hepatitis B.
d. T
e. F—A diagnosis of non-A, non-B hepatitis is made when there is no serological evidence of infection with hepatitis A, hepatitis B, cytomegalovirus or Epstein–Barr virus.

A.8.3
a. F—Relapses of hepatitis are rare but more common following hepatitis A and usually occur within 8 weeks of the initial presentation. They are precipitated by alcohol and exercise. Full recovery occurs.
b. F—Chronic liver disease is a complication of both hepatitis B and non-A, non-B hepatitis.
c. F—Men are two to three times more likely to become chronic carriers of hepatitis B.
d. T
e. T

A.8.4
a. T
b. F—Hepatitis A is spread by the faecal-oral route.
c. T
d. T
e. T

Q.8.5 Hepatitis A:

a. Is spread by the faecal-oral route
b. Is associated with a chronic carrier state in 5%–10% of cases
c. Has a long incubation period of 100 days
d. May be distinguished from hepatitis B and non-A, non-B hepatitis by the level of the aminotransferase enzymes
e. Is diagnosed by the presence of IgM-specific anti-hepatitis A virus (HAV) in the serum

Q.8.6 A patient who is found to carry hepatitis B surface antibody:

a. Is a carrier of hepatitis B
b. Is probably immune to hepatitis B
c. Requires vaccination against hepatitis B
d. Is infectious to others and may transmit hepatitis B
e. Should notify his dentist before any treatment can be performed

Q.8.7 Answer true or false:

a. Delta antigen is a transmissible agent requiring hepatitis B virus for its replication
b. The delta agent is a DNA virus
c. The delta antigen is associated with the RNA genome of the virus and is coated with HBs antigen
d. The delta antigen is common in Western homosexual men
e. The presence of the delta agent is associated with a more rapid progression to cirrhosis
f. Anti-d is detectable in the serum by a radioimmunoassay
g. The delta antigen cannot be detected in the serum in acute infection

For answers see over

A.8.5 a. T
b. F—Hepatitis B is associated with a chronic carrier state in 5%–10% of cases.
c. F—Hepatitis A has a short incubation period with a mean of 33 days.
d. F—The aminotransferase level does not distinguish between different forms of viral hepatitis.
e. T—The IgM-specific anti-HAV test is the diagnostic method of choice for hepatitis A.

A.8.6 a. F
b. T
c. F
d. F
e. F

Hepatitis B surface antibody is the protective antibody against reinfection.

A.8.7 a. T
b. F—It is an RNA virus.
c. T
d. F—It is uncommon.
e. T
f. T
g. F—Acute infection can in some cases be diagnosed by the demonstration of the delta antigen in the serum after cleavage of the hepatitis B surface antigen coat from the virus particle.

9. *Genital Herpes*

An Ode to Herpes

Primary herpes (genital) II,
Results in agonies in the loo,
Urine in the bladder retained,
(Neurogenic or vulva pained),
Only at first can the lesions last weeks,
Recurrences are only mild and meek,
"Acyclovir please", the patients all cry,
"Please give me a year's supply".

Doctors please take note of this,
Assess the lesions and *patient distress,*
Ask of their lives, the partner and job,
Do not the patients of counselling rob.

And please be nice to the PGLs,
They and the AIDs have herpes like hell,
With recurrences anal and penile too,
That last for weeks, at least a few,
Why no oral recurrences in AIDS please?
I'm afraid I cannot answer with ease.

"Remain free of herpes, how, what's new?
Monogamy only, or a durexed – – – –."

Q.9.1 Cytomegalovirus infection:

a. May cause a glandular fever-like disease
b. Is another cause of genital herpes
c. Causes haemorrhagic retinal exudates in the immunocompromised
d. May cause a colitis in the immunocompetent
e. Is a cause of acute hepatitis

Q.9.2 The following are antiviral drugs which are effective in the treatment of herpes simplex infections:

a. Alpha interferon
b. Acyclovir
c. Idoxuridine
d. Vinblastine
e. Vidarabine

Q.9.3 Answer true or false for these statements:

a. Seventy per cent of neonates born with HSV infection are born to mothers with no history of HSV infection
b. Women with genital HSV infection may shed virus from the cervix in the absence of vulval sores
c. A condom is no protection from sores on the glans penis as HSV can pass through rubber
d. Orofacial herpes is due to HSV 2 in 50% of cases
e. Contacts of genital HSV patients are traced by law in the United Kingdom

Q.9.4 The diagnosis of HSV infection may be confirmed by:

a. Light microscopy of a Gram-stained smear
b. Viral culture
c. Cytological examination using a Papanicolaou smear
d. Electron microscopy
e. Restriction endonuclease analysis

For answers see over

Answers

A.9.1
a. T
b. F—Genital herpes is caused by herpes simplex virus.
c. T—Haemorrhagic retinal exudates are characteristic of CMV retinitis. AIDS patients may have non-haemorrhagic exudates which are currently of uncertain aetiology.
d. T—Cytomegalovirus very rarely causes a colitis in the immunocompetent.
e. T

A.9.2
a. F
b. T
c. T
d. F
e. T

A.9.3
a. T
b. T
c. F
d. F—The correct answer is 20% (in most parts of the United Kingdom).
e. F

A.9.4
a. F
b. T
c. T—This is an insensitive diagnostic method.
d. T
e. T

Q.9.5 Consider the following statements about herpes simplex virus infections — which are true?

a. Genital HSV infection is associated with an increased risk of cervical carcinoma
b. In vitro acyclovir resistance can occur in both HSV I and II strains
c. No proven vaccine for the prevention of HSV infection is available
d. Neonatal HSV infection carries a 10% mortality
e. Fifty per cent of the DNA content of HSV II is similar to that in HSV I

Q.9.6 Common features of primary genital herpes simplex infection are:

a. Fever
b. Neck stiffness
c. Erythema marginatum
d. Dysuria in women
e. Hepatitis

Q.9.7 The differential diagnosis of genital HSV infection includes:

a. Behcet's disease
b. Scabies
c. Reiter's syndrome
d. Stevens–Johnson syndrome
e. Syphilis

For answers see over

A.9.5
a. T—No *causative* association has been shown between HSV and cervical cancer.
b. T
c. T
d. F—Fifty per cent mortality, even with treatment.
e. T

A.9.6
a. T
b. T
c. F—Erythema multiforme may occur.
d. T
e. F

A.9.7
a. T
b. T
c. T
d. T
e. T

Q.9.8 **A 24-year-old girl attends your clinic. She has culture-confirmed attacks of genital herpes that recur every 3–4 weeks. She tells you she cannot bring herself to tell her new boyfriend that she has "herpes" but that intercourse is imminent.**

She should be managed as follows:

a. She should be told to tell the boyfriend she has herpes
b. She should be told to break up with the boyfriend
c. Given a 6-month course of oral acyclovir in the first place to prevent recurrences
d. Given a 3-week course of oral acyclovir in the first place to prevent recurrences
e. Discuss with her why she finds it impossible to tell her boyfriend

Q.9.9 **Answer true or false about primary genital herpes:**

a. It is the same as first-attack genital herpes
b. It may result in a neurogenic bladder
c. It may lead to urinary retention because of severe vulval pain
d. Viral shedding time is reduced considerably by giving acyclovir
e. Recurrences are more likely after primary HSV I

Q.9.10 **In primary genital herpes simplex infection:**

a. Systemic symptoms are commoner in women
b. Unilateral lesions are commonly found
c. Virus may be isolated in culture from patients for 10 days (mean duration)
d. In women, cervical infection occurs in 25%
e. Inguinal lymphadenopathy is rare

Q.9.11 **The following are herpes viruses:**

a. Cytomegalovirus
b. Rabies
c. *Chlamydia trachomatis*
d. Varicella zoster
e. Epstein–Barr virus

For answers see over

A.9.8 a. F—This would be a value judgement imposed on the patient.
b. F—See a) above.
c. F—A shorter course of acyclovir might make her confident enough to tell the partner who may then feel that cessation of intercourse during recurrences is preferable to her going on long-term acyclovir.
d. T—See c) above.
e. T—Once this subject is broached her real anxieties and fears may be revealed.

A.9.9 a. F—First-attack genital herpes occurs when the patient has met HSV before (e.g. HSV I orally in the past; HSV II currently). Primary genital herpes is the first attack of any HSV.
b. T—Urinary retention may be due to reflex spasm or due to a neurogenic bladder.
c. T—See b) above.
d. T
e. F—HSV II primaries are more likely to recur.

A.9.10 a. T—Seventy per cent women versus 40% for men.
b. T
c. T
d. F—Over 80%.
e. F—Common >80%.

A.9.11 a. T
b. F
c. F
d. T
e. T

Q.9.12 The management of recurrent genital herpes includes:

a. Regular saline washes
b. Idoxuridine applications
c. Counselling of the patient
d. Acyclovir cream
e. Ultraviolet light therapy

Q.9.13 Genital herpes simplex infection in pregnancy:

a. Is associated with spontaneous abortion
b. Is associated with cleft palate of the fetus
c. Is associated with preterm labour
d. Always needs delivery by Caesarean section
e. Is said to result in a fatal disseminated infection in the *mother*

Q.9.14 Primary genital HSV infection:

a. May lead to aseptic meningitis
b. Can occur in patients with a history of cold sores
c. Has an incubation period of 14–21 days
d. May be painless
e. Is always due to HSV 2

For answers see over

A.9.12 a. T
b. F—These are expensive and clinically ineffective.
c. T
d. T—But success depends on starting treatment very early on in the attack.
e. F

A.9.13 a. T
b. F
c. T
d. F—If there are no lesions at term in the vulva or cervix and the membranes are intact, vaginal delivery may be allowed. Such a neonate should be closely followed for signs of neonatal herpes for a number of weeks.
e. T—Very rarely.

A.9.14 a. T
b. F
c. F—Two to 10 days
d. T—But this is very rare.
e. F—Eighty per cent due to HSV 2 in most parts of the United Kingdom.

10. *Human Immunodeficiency Virus (HIV)*[1] *Related Disease and Immunology*

1 HIV is the new internationally recognised name for HTLV III/LAV

HIV Virology/Transmission

Q.10.1 HIV is:

a. An RNA virus
b. Lipid enveloped
c. Sensitive to gamma irradiation
d. Inactivated by heating at 56°C for 30 min
e. Sensitive to a 1% solution of hypochlorite (household bleach)

Q.10.2 HIV:

a. Is the causative agent of adult T-cell leukaemia (ATCL) in some patients
b. Can be cultured in vitro in human T cells
c. Infects cells bearing the CD4 antigen
d. Can be differentiated from other retroviruses by the production of reverse transcriptase
e. Has been shown to infect monocytes and B cells in vitro

Q.10.3 HIV has been isolated from:

a. Whole blood
b. Plasma
c. Cell-free semen
d. CSF
e. Brain cells of infected individuals

Q.10.4 Antibodies to HIV:

a. Are strongly virus neutralising in asymptomatic carriers
b. Can be detected in the serum of >95% of patients with the acquired immune deficiency syndrome (AIDS)
c. Are always present in people found to be carrying viable HIV
d. Are only of IgG type
e. Serial titres predict the likelihood of developing full-blown AIDS

For answers see over

A.10.1 a. T
b. T—This means that the virus is susceptible to soaps and detergents.
c. F
d. T
e. T

A.10.2 a. F—HTLV I is the virus implicated in ATCL.
b. T—The usual means of isolation is by culturing in a virus-permissive T-cell line.
c. T—HIV infects cells via the surface antigen CD4, which acts as a receptor for the virus.
d. F—Retroviruses are RNA viruses characterised by their ability to make DNA copies of themselves. The enzyme used for this is reverse transcriptase and is found in all retroviruses.
e. T—Some monocytes and transformed B cells express the CD4 antigen and can therefore be infected.

A.10.3 a. T
b. T
c. T
d. T
e. T—HIV has been cultured from the brain cells of infected individuals. The cell of origin of the virus is at present not certain.

A.10.4 a. F—The antibodies that have been detected to HIV are either only very weakly virus neutralising or non-virus neutralising.
b. T
c. F—Both false positives and false negatives occur in all the antibody tests. Infected individuals may be negative in the early infection before antibody develops, or in the late stages of AIDS when antibody levels may fall due to severe immune suppression.
d. F—IgM antibodies are also produced especially in the early stages of infection.
e. F—There is no correlation.

Q.10.5 HIV has been shown to be transmitted by:

a Heterosexual (vaginal) intercourse
b. Transplacentally
c. Breast milk
d. Aerosols of contaminated body fluid
e. Use of HIV-contaminated swimming pools/jacuzzis

Q.10.6 Infection with HIV:

a. Is asymptomatic in the majority of individuals
b. May persist in an asymptomatic form for >5 years
c. May be associated with an acute self-limiting illness consisting of fever, lymphadenopathy, rash and myalgia
d. Is a cause of thrombocytopenia
e. Often causes hilar lymphadenopathy

Epidemiology of HIV Infection

Q.10.7 Risk groups for AIDS include:

a. Intravenous drug abusers
b. Blood donors
c. Female sexual partners of bisexual men
d. Mentally handicapped children
e. Central Africans

Q.10.8 In the acquired immune deficiency syndrome (AIDS):

a. Cases were first reported in the United States in 1981
b. The doubling time for reported cases in the United States was 3 months in the first 2 years of the epidemic
c. Greater than 60% of cases present with Kaposi's sarcoma
d. In central African cases the ratio of male to female cases is about 1.2:1
e. The incidence of Kaposi's sarcoma is higher in haemophiliacs with AIDS than in the other risk groups

For answers see over

A.10.5 a. T
b. T
c. T
d. F
e. F—HIV is spread by three main routes, sexually, either homosexual or heterosexual, via blood and its products and transplacentally. There is no evidence for aerosol, salivary or water-borne transmission.

A.10.6 a. T
b. T
c. T—This mild illness usually occurs around the time of seroconversion, but only in a minority of infected individuals.
d. T—Many individuals who are HIV infected will develop thromboctopenia at some stage. This is thought to be mediated by immune complexes.
e. F—Hilar lymphadenopathy due to HIV is exceptional; its presence usually indicates opportunistic infection or lymphoma.

A.10.7 a. T—Through sharing needles, syringes, etc. contaminated with infected blood.
b. F—There is no danger in blood *donation*.
c. T—HIV is transmitted heterosexually via vaginal and anal intercourse.
d. F
e. T—There is a high carriage rate of HIV and AIDS in most central African countries.

A.10.8 a. T
b. F—The doubling rate in both the United States and the United Kingdom in the first 3 years of the epidemic was 6–8 months.
c. F—Kaposi's sarcoma is the presenting feature in approximately 30% of homosexual men with AIDS, and far less than this in haemophiliacs and AIDS acquired through blood transfusion.
d. T—In Africa AIDS has always been a heterosexual disease.
e. F—See c).

Persistent Generalised Lymphadenopathy

Q.10.9 To be classified as having persistent generalised lymphadenopathy (PGL) a patient must meet the following criteria:

a. Have generalised lymphadenopathy for at least 12 months
b. Have lymphadenopathy at more than one extrainguinal site
c. Lymph nodes must be greater than 1 cm in diameter
d. Have weight loss of at least 10% of total body weight over the preceding 3 months
e. Have persistent depletion of T-helper lymphocytes

Q.10.10 Persistent generalised lymphadenopathy:

a. Is a cause of lymphoedema
b. May spontaneously resolve
c. Is commonly unilateral
d. Shows diagnostic features on histology
e. Commonly resolves around the time of the first opportunist infection in patients who develop AIDS

Q.10.11 Poor prognostic features for progression to AIDS in patients with PGL include:

a. Lymph nodes at > four sites
b. Recurrence of herpes zoster, i.e. shingles
c. Hilar lymphadenopathy
d. Macroscopic oral candidiasis
e. Recurrent episodes of gonorrhoea

For answers see over

A.10.9 a. F
b. T
c. T
d. F
e. F

The definition of PGL is lymphadenopathy of greater than 1 cm diameter in more than one extrainguinal site for more than 3 months for which no other cause can be found. No laboratory criteria are required. This is an HIV-related condition, and a percentage of affected individuals will eventually develop AIDS.

A.10.10 a. F
b. T—But rarely.
c. F
d. F—Routine histology usually shows a non-specific picture of reactive hyperplasia.
e. T

A.10.11 a. F—The number of sites does not correlate with prognosis.
b. T—This may be an early sign of immune dysfunction and precede opportunist infection by several months.
c. F—This is not a feature of PGL.
d. T—In the absence of other causes, e.g. antibiotic use or diabetes, this is indicative of immune deficiency.
e. F—Although numerous episodes of infection including STD may increase the likelihood of developing AIDS due to persistent viral activation (when T cells are activated so is the virus); however, recurrent episodes are not a bad prognostic sign and do not indicate immune deficiency.

N.B. The group of symptoms and signs including persistent weight loss, fevers and night sweats, diarrhoea, oral candida, chronic ulcerative herpes simplex and leucopenia are sometimes termed "prodromal AIDS" or AIDS-related complex (ARC) and represent a group of patients with HIV infection who have a high chance of progressing to full-blown AIDS.

Q.10.12 Histology/immunohistology of a lymph node biopsy from a patient with PGL may show:

a. Germinal centre hyperplasia
b. Depletion of the B-cell areas
c. HIV viral particles in the follicular dendritic cells
d. HIV viral particles in the lymphocytes of the paracortical areas
e. Invasion of "suppressor" (CD 8) lymphocytes into the germinal centres

A medical student named Bell,
Rang out "About PGL,
I know that the causes
In humans, not horses,
are HELOT, CMV and Brucell(osis)".

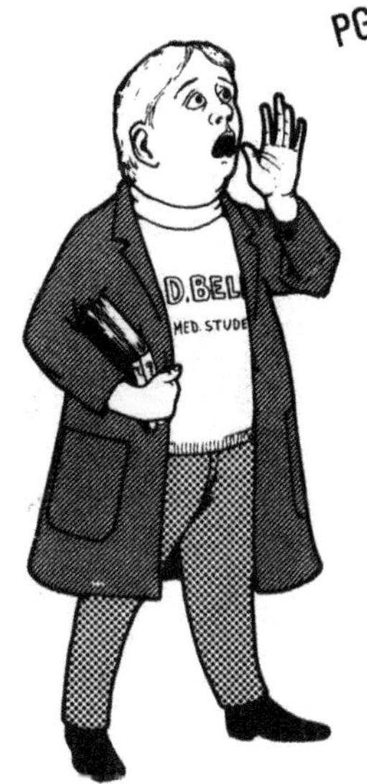

The differential diagnosis of PGL in young people is:

H — HIV infection
E — EB virus
L — Lymphomas
O — Other (e.g. toxoplasmosis, syphilis)
T — TB

Cytomegalovirus (CMV) is another cause of PGL, as is brucellosis if there is a history of intake of unpasteurised milk.

A.10.12 a. T
b. F
c. T—Most of the virus particles within lymph nodes are found in the phagocytic and antigen-presenting follicular dendritic cells rather than in the lymphocytes, which either do not contain virus or do not express it.
d. F—See c).
e. T—This is a typical finding, though not specific.

Clinical Manifestations of HIV Infection

Q.10.13 Which of the following criteria have to be met before a diagnosis of AIDS can be made:

a. A positive HIV antibody test
b. Demonstration of viable HIV in the blood or other body fluid
c. The confirmed diagnosis of an opportunist infection or tumour indicative of a defect in cell-mediated immunity in a person with no other cause for immunosuppression
d. Persistent depletion of T-helper lymphocytes
e. A persistently inverted T-helper/suppressor ratio

Q.10.14 Neurological manifestations of AIDS and HIV infection include:

a. Generalised cerebral atrophy
b. Personality changes
c. CNS lymphoma
d. Increased incidence of multiple sclerosis
e. Cerebral toxocariasis

Q.10.15 Gastrointestinal infections seen in association with AIDS include:

a. *Salmonella typhimurium*
b. Cryptococcosis
c. Cryptosporidiosis
d. Cytomegalovirus colitis
e. Oesophageal candidiasis

For answers see over

A.10.13 a. F
b. F
c. T
d. F
e. F

AIDS is a clinical diagnosis based on the finding of an opportunist infection or tumour indicative of a defect in cell-mediated immunity in an individual who has no reason to be immunosuppressed, i.e. is not on any immunosuppressive therapy and does not have a tumour to account for this.

A.10.14 a. T—Due to direct HIV infection.
b. T—Due to direct HIV infection or to opportunist infection.
c. T—This has an increased incidence in AIDS patients and is usually of B-cell origin.
d. F—Although it has been suggested that multiple sclerosis is a retroviral disease there is no increase in AIDS/HIV infection.
e. F—Toxoplasmosis is the common finding.

A.10.15 a. T—Most bacteria are not a major problem as they are extracellular and eradicated by the humoral immune system. However, salmonella is a facultative intracellular organism and therefore an intact cell-mediated system is necessary for its elimination.
b. F—Cryptococcus commonly causes meningitis and occasionally lung infection but not gut symptoms.
c. T—Cryptosporidiosis is primarily a disease of fowl and young cattle. In immunocompetent humans it causes a self-limiting diarrhoea, but in immunocompromised individuals the diarrhoea is severe and watery and may be fatal. There is no effective antimicrobial agent against this organism.
d. T—Cytomegalovirus causes a picture very similar to ulcerative colitis, which in severe cases leads on to toxic megacolon.
e. T—This causes severe burning dysphagia, but usually responds to treatment with ketoconazole.

Q.10.16 Skin conditions with an increased frequency in patients with HIV infection include:

a. Seborrhoeic dermatitis
b. Folliculitis
c. Vasculitis
d. Erythema nodosum
e. Erythema multiforme

Q.10.17 Infections seen commonly in patients with AIDS include:

a. Perianal herpes simplex
b. Molluscum contageosum
c. *Legionella*
d. Listeriosis
e. Brucellosis

Q.10.18 Patients with AIDS have an increased incidence of the following tumours:

a. Non-Hodgkins lymphoma
b. Carcinoma of the penis
c. Bowen's sarcoma
d. Kaposi's sarcoma of lymph nodes
e. Hepatocellular carcinoma

For answers see over

A.10.16 a. T—In some cases this is due to a fungal infection.
b. T—Often no organism is isolated.
c. T
d. F
e. F

A.10.17 a. T—Chronic ulcerative perianal HSV occurs in approximately 75% of homosexual AIDS patients. Urethral and oral HSV is less of a problem.
b. T—Particularly on the face.
c. F—Surprisingly this infection does not have increased incidence in this group of patients
d. F—As for c).
e. F

A.10.18 a. T—Particularly B-cell lymphomas, which are thought to be Epstein–Barr virus linked.
b. F
c. F
d. T—If there is cutaneous Kaposi's sarcoma then there is nearly always lymph node involvement.
e. F—Although there is an increased rate of hepatitis B carriers in the HIV-infected group, there is no evidence yet of an increased incidence of hepatocellular carcinoma.

Q.10.19 ***Pneumocystis carinii* pneumonia (PCP) usually presents with:**

a Persistent productive cough
b. A history of 2–4 weeks of increasing shortness of breath
c. Fever of >37.5°C
d. Decrease in arterial PO_2 with normal arterial PCO_2 and transfer factor
e. Perihilar interstitial shadowing on chest X-ray with sparing of the apical and supradiaphragmatic areas

For answers see over

A.10.19 a. F—The cough of PCP is characteristically non-productive.
b. T
c. T
d. F—*Pneumocystis carinii* pneumonia is an alveolar disease and is associated with a decreased transfer of gases across the membrane, causing a lowered PO_2 and transfer factor. The greater diffusability of CO_2 allows this to remain normal.
e. T

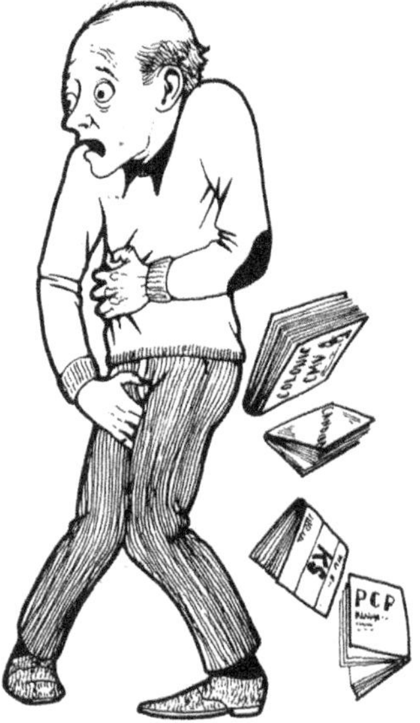

A hypochondriac bald-headed swot,
Said, "I know I've got the damn lot",
Colonic CMV,
Candida, *KS, PCP,*
And they're caused by "T" helper cell rot.

AIDS patients commonly present with PCP colonic CMV or KS. The basic immunological defect in AIDS is "T" helper cell defect.

Q.10.20 In Kaposi's sarcoma (KS) in patients with AIDS:

a. The lesions are usually pruritic
b. The tumour never matastasises
c. Epstein–Barr virus DNA is nearly always found within the tumour cells
d. The patients with KS but no opportunist infections and a normal lymphocyte count have an 80% chance of surviving 2 years
e. The number of lesions tends to increase during periods of opportunist infection

Paediatric AIDS

Q.10.21 If a pregnant women is found to be infected with HIV:

a. She has approximately a 50% chance of infecting her child
b. She will be likely to develop more severe disease herself during the pregnancy
c. Caesarian section would ensure that the fetus was not infected
d. There would be an increased chance of congenital neurological defects in the child
e. A second pregnancy would carry the same risk of infection to the fetus

Q.10.22 The common presenting features of AIDS in children infected transplacentally/perinatally are:

a. Lymphocytic pneumonitis
b. Failure to thrive
c. Parotitis
d. Atopic eczema
e. Presentation at 2–2½ years

For answers see over

A.10.20 a. F
b. T—Kaposi's sarcoma is multifocal in origin and does not metastasise.
c. F—The DNA of cytomegalovirus may be found within some KS tumours.
d. T—This is the best prognostic group within the AIDS diagnosis.
e. T—This may reflect either the decrease in immune status that allows an opportunist infection to occur or the immunosuppressive effect of the infection itself.

A.10.21 a. T
b. T—This may be due to the allogeneic stimulation of the fetus or to the general decreased immune function observed during pregnancy.
c. F—The infection is usually passed transplacentally at an early stage of gestation.
d. T—There is an increased risk of microcephaly.
e. T—HIV infection persists for several years and possibly for life and therefore can be transmitted in further pregnancies.

A.10.22 a. T—This is much more common in children with AIDS than adults and is due to proliferation of CD8+ (suppressor) lymphocytes in response to Epstein–Barr virus infection.
b. T
c. T—Another feature which is much more common in children.
d. T
e. F—Children may present at this age but it is usually at 6–9 months that problems develop in infants infected during pregnancy.

Treatment

Q.10.23 The following compounds are active against the corresponding organism/infection:

a. Activated glutaraldehyde — *Cryptosporidium*
b. Sulphadiazine + pyrimethamine — cerebral toxoplasmosis
c. Trimethoprim + sulphonamide — *Pneumocystis carinii*
d. Intravenous miconazole — cryptococcal meningitis
e. Isoprinosine — oesophageal candidiasis

Q.10.24 The following drugs have been shown to have activity against HIV in vitro:

a. Interferon alpha
b. Interleukin-1
c. Interleukin-2
d. Suramin
e. DHPG [9-(1,3-dihydroxy, 2-propoxy methyl)guanine]

Immunology of HIV Infection

Q.10.25 Immunological testing of patients with AIDS usually shows:

a. Decrease in the total number of CD4+ lymphocytes
b. Increase in the total number of CD8+ lymphocytes
c. Hypogammaglobulinaemia
d. Increased spontaneous immunoglobulin production by B cells in vitro
e. Decreased reactivity in delayed-type hypersensitivity skin tests to previously encountered antigen

For answers see over

A.10.23 a. F—None of the commonly used antiseptics/sterilising agents are effective.
b. T
c. T—Used in high dose.
d. F—The treatment of choice for cryptococcal meningitis is a 4-week course of intravenous flucytosine and amphoteracin B followed by 2 weeks of oral flucytosine.
e. F—Ketoconazole is the drug used for oesophageal candidiasis.
Isoprinosine is an antiviral and immunomodulating drug used in herpes simplex infection and is also being tried as a measure to prevent HIV-infected patients developing AIDS.

A.10.24 a. T—Alpha-interferon is a non-specific antiviral agent.
b. F—Interleukin-1 is a monocyte/macrophage product that stimulates lymphocytes but is not directly active against viruses.
c. F—Interleukin-2 is a lymphocyte product (lymphokine) sometimes called T-cell growth factor that stimulates other lymphocytes but again is not directly active against viruses.
d. T
e. F—DHPG is an acyclovir-like drug that has shown activity against cytomegalovirus.

A.10.25 a. T
b. F—In AIDS patients the total CD8+ (suppressor) lymphocyte numbers are normal although the percentage may be raised. The total numbers may be raised early in HIV infection.
c. F—Characteristically there is a polyclonal increase in immunoglobulins.
d. T—This may account for the increase in serum immunoglobulins.
e. T—This is a characteristic finding.

Q.10.26 Patients with AIDS:

a. Have increased levels of immune complexes in the serum
b. About 50% develop a maculopapular rash when treated with Septrin (cotrimoxazole)
c. Are able to produce antibodies to neoantigens but not to antigens that have been encountered previously
d. Have abnormal monocyte/macrophage function
e. Have normal natural killer cell function

General Immunology

Q.10.27 T cells:

a. Are morphologically distinguishable from B cells
b. Subsets containing different functional groups can be determined using monoclonal antibodies (McAbs) to cell surface antigens
c. The phenotype described by the McAbs to the CD8 antigen includes the T cells involved in delayed-type hypersensitivity (DTH) reactions
d. Recognise foreign antigen only when presented in the context of MHC antigens
e. Cytotoxic T cells are involved in the destruction of virally infected cells

Q.10.28 B cells:

a. Can be detected by the presence of surface immunoglobulin
b. Only produce immunoglobulin of one light chain type at one time
c. Proliferate in response to mitogens
d. Can produce antibody in the absence of T-cell help
e. Are mostly found in the paracortical areas of the lymph nodes

For answers see over

A.10.26 a. T
b. T—Approximately 50%–60% will have this complication.
c. F—It is the new antigen that AIDS patients are unable to respond to.
d. T—This may be due to direct infection with HIV or to blockade of the Fc receptors by immune complexes which are necessary for efficient attachment and ingestion of microorganisms.
e. F—Natural killer cells are thought to play an important role in "immunological surveillance" and tumour recognition. In AIDS both numbers and function of these cells are depressed and may be partly responsible for the increased incidence of tumours.

A.10.27 a. F
b. T—McAbs to detect CD4+ lymphocytes (helper/inducer), CD8+ (suppressor/cytotoxic) and other groups are commonly used. However, although these phenotypes usually correspond to the function listed here there are exceptions, i.e. where a CD4+ cell in fact has suppressor function.
c. F—The T cells involved in DTH belong to the CD4+ subset (see above).
d. T—This is a characteristic feature of T cells. Foreign antigen will not be recognised unless it is presented with either a HLA Class I (for suppressor/cytotoxic T cells) or II antigen (helper T cells).
e. T—These are the most important cells in the elimination of cell-associated virus.

A.10.28 a. T—All mature B cells carry immunoglobulin of the class that they are destined to make. This is present on the cell surface, with the antigen-binding site facing outwards to act as the antigen receptor.
b. T
c. T
d. T—Usually T-cell help is required for antibody production but some antigens, e.g. polysaccharides, are T-cell independent and B cells can respond directly.
e. F—The germinal centre contains most of the B cells.

Q.10.29 Complement:

a. C3b component is one of the major opsonins
b. Deficiencies are associated with an increased susceptibility to disseminated neisserial infections
c. Can be activated directly by bacterial cell walls
d. Components are raised as part of the acute-phase response
e. Fixation tests are often used to detect antibodies to herpes simplex virus

Q.10.30 Cell-mediated immunity is thought to play an important part in the eradication of the following organisms:

a. Mycobacteria
b. Herpesviruses
c. *Salmonella*
d. *Listeria*
e. *Brucella*

Q.10.31 Macrophages:

a. Produce interleukin-2
b. Express DR antigen
c. Are activated by interferon gamma
d. Show immunological memory for previously encountered antigen
e. Contain the enzyme myeloperoxidase

Q.10.32 Alpha interferons:

a. Are species specific, virus non-specific
b. Are produced within 6 h of viral infection
c. React with a cell membrane receptor
d. Suppresses natural killer cell activity
e. Are normally acid labile

For answers see over

A.10.29 a. T—C3b and IgG are the most important opsonins.
b. T
c. T—Via the alternative pathway.
d. T
e. T—When antibody and antigen are combined, immune complexes result which activate complement.

A.10.30
a.-e. T—These are all intracellular pathogens and cell-mediated immunity therefore plays the most important role.

A.10.31 a. F—Interleukin-2 is only produced by lymphocytes. Interleukin-1 is the monocyte/macrophage product.
b. T—DR antigen is a class II HLA antigen and essential for efficient presentation of foreign antigen to CD4+ (helper) T cells.
c. T—Interferon gamma is a lymphokine which is thought one of the most important macrophage-activating factors.
d. F
e. T

A.10.32 a. T
b. T
c. T—There is a specific receptor for interferons on cell surfaces.
d. F—Characteristically they enhance NK cell activity.
e. F—Characteristically alpha and beta interferons (viral IFNO) are acid stable and this differentiates them from interferon gamma (immune IFN) which is acid labile. In AIDS an unusual acid-labile alpha interferon is present in the serum in large amounts.

Q.10.33 Immune complexes:

a. Can be detected in the blood of healthy individuals
b. Activate complement via the alternative pathway
c. Can be detected in the serum by the ability to bind C1q
d. Only activate complement if the antibody is of IgM type
e. Are a cause of thrombocytopenia

Q.10.34 In the immune response to viral infection:

a. Antibodies can only neutralise extracellular virus
b. Interferon alpha is directly viricidal
c. Cytotoxic T cells can only recognise viral antigen when presented with class 1 antigen
d. Viral antigens are usually expressed in the cell cytoplasm but not on the cell surface
e. Natural killer cells non-specifically destroy virally infected cells

Q.10.35 Delayed-type hypersensitivity skin tests:

a. Show greatest reaction at 12–24 h
b. Are a test of macrophage function
c. To purified protein derivative (ppd) is often positive in patients with sarcoid even if they have not been immunised with BCG
d. 0.1 ml ppd at 1 in 1000 would be a suitable dose in a patient suspected of having tuberculosis
e. Streptokinase would be a suitable antigen to test for general cell-mediated immunity

Q.10.36 Immunoglobulins:

a. IgA is produced by epithelial cells
b. IgG_1 and G_3 are important in immunity to encapsulated organisms
c. IgG in secretions is totally derived from plasma
d. IgA deficiency can be found in 1 in 500 healthy blood donors
e. IgD is only found on the surface of immature B cells

For answers see over

A.10.33 a. T—After eating, immune complexes are commonly found circulating in the blood.
b. F—Via the classical pathway.
c. T
d. F—IgG antibody in immune complexes can also activate complement.
e. T—Immune complexes can bind via the Fc portion of the IgG within them to the Fc receptors on platelets and the platelets are then taken up by the reticuloendothelial system.

A.10.34 a. T
b. F—Interferon acts by preventing the infection of uninfected cells and by reducing virus production in infected cells.
c. T
d. F—Viral antigens are expressed both on the cell surface and in the cytoplasm.
e. T

A.10.35 a. F—The maximum reaction is usually at 48–72 h.
b. T—Both macrophages and lymphocytes need to be functioning for a positive DTH.
c. F—Patients with sarcoid are characteristically negative to DTH with ppd.
d. F—This is the dose to test for anergy in an individual without TB. A patient with TB is likely to respond to a much lower dose and would have a very severe reaction to 1:1000.
e. T—Streptokinase and *Candida albicans* are antigens that most individuals have been exposed to and would be expected to react positively in DTH.

A.10.36 a. F—IgA is produced mainly by plasma cells in the mucosae; however, it is excreted by epithelial cells.
b. F—IgG_{2+4} are the important ones.
c. F—IgG is also secreted locally.
d. T—IgA deficiency is usually asymptomatic.
e. T—It is lost as the cell matures.

11. *Pelvic Inflammatory Disease*

Q.11.1 The following can be described as pelvic inflammatory disease (PID):

a. Pelvic peritonitis
b. Salpingo-oophoritis
c. Cervicitis
d. Endometritis
e. Urethritis

Q.11.2 Recognised long-term sequelae of PID include:

a. Chronic pelvic pain
b. Tubal infertility
c. Recurrent early pregnancy loss
d. Increased risk of ectopic pregnancy
e. Anovulatory cycles

Q.11.3 In a patient with lower abdominal pain, clinical features that support a diagnosis of PID are:

a. Pyrexia
b. Unilateral lower abdominal pain
c. Hb less than 10 g/litre
d. Serum β-human chorionic gonadotrophin (BHCG) greater than 400 units
e. Purulent cervical discharge

For answers see over

Answers

A.11.1 a. T
b. T
c. F
d. T
e. F

The term PID is used to describe an infection of the upper female genital tract. The division between upper and lower genital tract is the cervix; thus any infection at or below the cervix is a lower genital tract infection.

A.11.2 a. T
b. T
c. F
d. T
e. F

Chronic lower abdominal pain is sometimes a result of pelvic infection and this is not always due to reinfection. Infertility after PID is due to tubal damage, which in turn leads to increased risk of ectopic pregnancy. The menstrual cycle is not affected and the cause of recurrent early pregnancy loss has yet to be established, although postendometritis intrauterine adhesions have been suggested.

A.11.3 a. T—Fever may occur but is less pronounced in ectopic pregnancy or painful ovarian cysts.
b. F—More common with an ectopic pregnancy.
c. F—See b) above.
d. F—See b) above.
e. T—Pelvic inflammatory disease may also occur without any cervical discharge.

Q.11.4 Answer true or false:

a. Pelvic inflammatory disease is sexually transmitted
b. Eighty per cent of women with gonorrhoea develop salpingitis
c. A regime of penicillin and metronidazole (i.v.) is sufficient for most cases of PID
d. Bed rest and attention to general health is important in the management of PID
e. Pelvic inflammatory disease is rare in pregnancy

Q.11.5 Agents known to be responsible for acute salpingitis are:

a. *Trichomonas vaginalis*
b. *Gardnerella vaginalis*
c. *Esherichia coli*
d. Staphylococci
e. *Chlamydia trachomatis*

Q.11.6 Factors predisposing to an increased risk of acquiring acute salpingitis include:

a. Use of oral contraceptive pill
b. Frequent change of sexual partners
c. Previous episode of bacterial vaginosis
d. Previous tubal surgery
e. Age greater than 35 years

For answers see over

A.11.4 a. T—The most common known agents causing PID are both sexually transmitted — *Chlamydia trachomatis* and *Neisseria gonorrhoea*. It is very rare in women who are not sexually active, so must be considered to be sexually transmitted.
b. F—Only 10% of women with cervical gonorrhoea develop ascending infection.
c. F—Penicillin and metronidazole would probably successfully treat many cases of gonorrhoea and anaerobic bacteria but this regime does not cover *Chlamydia trachomatis*.
d. T
e. T

A.11.5 a. F
b. F
c. T
d. T
e. T

A.11.6 a. F—The oral contraceptive is thought to be protective.
b. T
c. F—Previous vaginal infections are not relevant.
d. T—It is thought that damaged fallopian tubes are more easily infected.
e. F—The age range for maximum incidence is 20–24 years.

12. *Prostatitis*

Q.12.1 Chronic low-grade pain in the perineum associated with finding clumps of pus (white) cells in expressed prostatic fluid and no significant bacterial growth in urine can be called:

a. Chronic bacterial prostatitis
b. Prostatodynia
c. Chronic non-bacterial prostatitis
d. Hypochondriasis
e. A psychosomatic pain

Q.12.2 The following are true about prostatic fluid obtained by digital massage of the prostate gland:

a. It is more easily obtained when the patient has not ejaculated for a week rather than a day or two ago
b. Even though it is uncomfortable, it is a safe procedure
c. It can be distinguished from urine by its colour and consistency
d. It may contain pus cells in the absence of symptoms
e. If *Chlamydia trachomatis* is present, it is best confirmed by cell culture

Q.12.3 Chronic prostatitis may be diagnosed by finding one or more of the following:

a. Clumps of white cells in expressed prostatic fluid
b. Coliform bacteria in expressed prostatic fluid
c. Pain produced by per rectal digital palpation of the prostate
d. Finding coliforms in a mid-stream urine specimen (MSU)
e. Finding *Staphylococcus albus* in a postprostatic massage urine in a concentration 1000 times greater than a premassage urine on three separate occasions

For answers see over

Answers

A.12.1 a. F
b. F
c. T
d. F
e. F

A.12.2 a. T—Presumably because of the build-up of fluid in the gland and vesicles.
b. F—It not uncommonly is a cause of severe vasovagal attacks.
c. T—It is white and viscous.
d. T
e. F—Prostatic fluid is toxic to the cell culture system normally used.

A.12.3 a. T—Prostatitis is said to be present when clumps of white (pus) cells are found in expressed prostatic fluid.
b. F—Finding coliforms in expressed prostatic fluid may reflect no more than contamination of prostatic fluid by urethral meatal commensal organisms. It, however, may reflect a prostatitis.
c. F—Digital examination of the prostate is, at the very least, uncomfortable even in normal patients. Conversely, patients with prostatitis may find prostatic massage a painless manoeuvre.
d. F—Coliforms in an MSU indicate a urinary tract infection. They give no clue to the presence or absence of prostatitis.
e. T—Urine samples obtained after prostatic massage can be compared to premassage urines. Where the concentration of organisms is ten times greater or more in the postprostatic urine compared with the preprostatic urine, it is assumed prostatitis is present, even if the organisms are generally considered non-pathogens (e.g. *Staphylococcus albus*).

Q.12.4 The following statements about acute prostatitis are true:

a. It is rarely seen in VD clinics
b. It is commonly caused by the gonococcus or enteric bacteria
c. It may present as a purulent discharge per rectum
d. The patient is often afebrile but has a moderate degree of prostatic pain
e. It usually responds to high doses of ampicillin/amoxicillin

Q.12.5 Chronic prostatic pain is usually felt in one or more of the following areas:

a. Perineum
b. Both renal angles
c. Suprapubic
d. Lower back (lumbosacral areas)
e. Lateral aspect of the thighs

Q.12.6 Which of the following antibiotics penetrate into the prostate:

a. Ampicillin
b. Cotrimoxazole
c. Doxycycline
d. Erythromycin
e. Penicillin G

For answers see over

A.12.4 a. T—Acute prostatitis is rarely seen in VD clinics and is most uncommon altogether since the advent of the antibiotic era.
b. T—Enteric bacteria (faecal streptococci, coliforms) and *Neisseria gonorrhoea* are the usual bacterial causes.
c. T—A prostatic abscess may burst into the urethra or rectum.
d. F—The patients have high swinging temperatures and great pain in the prostatic and perineal area.
e. T—Treatment is by bedrest, fluid replacement, analgesia and high-dose antibiotics; bacterial culture of an MSU will yield the bacteria for sensitivities. Amoxicillin or ampicillin in high dose will usually result in eradication of the infection.

A.12.5 a. T
b. F
c. T
d. T
e. F

Whatever the cause of the prostatic pain, patient's symptoms are consistently confined to certain areas. The pain may thus be felt in one or more of the following areas: perineum, lower back (lumbosacral), suprapubic area or medial aspect of the thigh.

A.12.6 a. F
b. T
c. T
d. T
e. F

13. *Psychological and Sexual Problems*

Q.13.1 Detectable anxiety and depression:

a. Are found in about a third of VD clinic patients
b. Are probably associated with frequent recurrences of genital herpes
c. May be the cause for night sweats, weight loss, shortness of breath, diarrhoea and headaches in an HIV antibody-positive homosexual who has PGL
d. Are found more commonly than expected by chance in patients with prostatodynia
e. Should be managed with diazepam regularly until the condition subsides

Q.13.2 The following are common causes of penile erectile failures:

a. Craniopharyngioma
b. Diabetes mellitus
c. Tricyclic antidepressants
d. Not being sexually attracted by the partner
e. Physical exhaustion

Q.13.3 The following are accepted treatments for premature ejaculation:

a. Clomipramine
b. Thioridazine (melleril)
c. Fantasising the actual partner as someone far more sexually exciting than the real partner
d. Will power
e. Lignocaine gel applied to the penis 10 min before intercourse

For answers see over

Answers

A.13.1 a. T—Using the General Health Questionnaire (GHQ), up to 40% of patients attending VD clinics in the United Kingdom have significant non-psychotic psychiatric illness.

b. T—The shorter the time between the first attack and first recurrence, the more likely a high GHQ score.

c. T—Anxiety and depression may cause all of the symptoms but they need organic investigation too.

d. T—Prostatodynia means painful prostate, with no evidence of malignancy or inflammation. Such patients are likely to have a higher GHQ score than controls.

e. F—Diazepam taken regularly for 4–6 weeks may result in physical dependency.

A.13.2 a. F—This is a rare cause of erectile failure (secondary to pressure effects on the pituitary fossa).

b. T—Diabetes mellitus particularly when poorly controlled is a common cause of erectile failure.

c. T—These drugs are still commonly prescribed for depressive illnesses.

d. T—People may stay in relationships after sexual attraction has ceased. In this case, erectile failure is not inappropriate.

e. T—In this situation, it is appropriate for erection to fail, particularly when tiredness is overwhelming.

A.13.3 a. T—This drug may control premature ejaculation.

b. T—See a) above.

c. F—A high level of sexual excitement contributes to premature ejaculation in young men. This treatment will thus make things worse.

d. F—Will power may help retard ejaculation (inconsistently) but usually results in lack of enjoyment for the man.

e. F—Lignocaine gel may initially be successful by reducing sensory input to the penis. This, however, is a marked skin sensitiser and the patient should anyway not become reliant on it. The squeeze technique is a successful non-pharmacological method of controlling premature ejaculation.

Q.13.4 A 35-year-old man has been seen in a clinic 10 times in 3 weeks. He has no physical abnormality and serological tests for syphilis are negative. He has a fixed idea that he has syphilis and requests treatment for his supposed infection. No amount of reassurance or explanation will shake this belief. He is an otherwise pleasant normal man.

The following facts are likely to be true about him:

a. He has an obsessional illness
b. He has a monosymptomatic delusion
c. He should be given a course of penicillin (benzathine penicillin 2.4 MU i.m.)
d. Successful management entails referral of the patient to a psychiatrist
e. He should be treated in the VD clinic with a low dose of pimozide in the first place

Q.13.5 A 27-year-old heterosexual man comes to a VD clinic complaining that he has acquired AIDS. He is anxious and depressed about this. He has run no risk at all of acquiring HIV virus apart from saying he picked it up from a toilet seat 1 year ago. He seems a pleasant but worried man, who in a way understands the illogicality of his belief, but cannot get away from these thoughts. You see him twice to reassure him and explain the facts to him but he remains worried and you can only temporarily reassure him.

The HIV antibody is negative.

The following are likely to be true about him:

a. He is deluded
b. He needs further explanation and reassurance
c. He needs pimozide plus psychotherapy
d. He is obsessional
e. He needs clomipramine plus psychotherapy

For answers see over

A.13.4 a. F—This man cannot be persuaded he has no illness even for a short time. He, therefore, has a delusion not an obsession. It is monosymptomatic because there are no other signs of a psychotic illness.
b. T—See a) above.
c. F—His requests for penicillin would continue after such treatment and would only confirm this incorrect diagnosis in his mind.
d. F—This patient would not see his problem as mental, rather organic and may, therefore, refuse to see a psychiatrist.
e. T—The appropriate treatment is pimozide.

A.13.5 a. F—He is not deluded as he can be reassured, even though only temporarily.
b. F—If explanation and reassurance have not been successful in two sessions, it is unlikely to succeed.
c. F—Pimozide is used in the control of monosymptomatic delusions.
d. T—The ruminations, with a certain degree of insight, strongly suggest he is obsessional.
e. T—Clomipramine is a tricyclic antidepressant that is very useful in patients with obsessional illnesses plus depression. It should be used in conjunction with psychotherapy, e.g. cognitive therapy.

14. *Syphilis*

Q.14.1 A clinical specimen to detect *Treponema pallidum* by dark-ground microscopy is best obtained by:

a. Gently rolling a cotton wool swab over the ulcer and transferring the material into saline on a microscope slide
b. Only taking dark-field specimens from painless lesions
c. Giving the patient a little gentle antiseptic (e.g. dilute Savlon) to use on the lesion a day before dark fields are attempted to facilitate clearing of other spirochaetes that might make differential diagnosis difficult
d. Abrading the lesion with gauze soaked in saline until it bleeds. It is then left to coagulate after which the resulting serum is lifted off with a coverslip and transferred directly to the microscope slide.
e. Giving the patient 250 mg penicillin V orally: 24 h later *T. pallidum* will swell up and will be more easily identifiable

Q.14.2 The differential diagnosis of general paresis of the insane (GPI) includes:

a. Anxiety state
b. Schizophrenia
c. Personality disorder
d. Endogenous depression
e. Mania

Q.14.3 The following are usually found in GPI:

a. Positive fluorescent treponemal antibody test (FTA) antibodies in the CSF
b. Cerebrovascular endarteritis
c. Cerebral atrophy
d. Hyperreflexia with upgoing plantars
e. Argyll–Robertson pupils

Q.14.4 Secondary syphilis is known to cause:

a. Generalised lymphadenopathy
b. Uveitis
c. Cardiomyopathy
d. Gummata of bone
e. The "sign of the groove"

For answers see over

Answers

A.14.1 a. F—All if not most of the serum will in this case be absorbed onto the swab so that none will be available for microscopy.

b. F—Rarely early syphilitic lesions are *painful*.

c. F—Antiseptics kill *T. pallidum* and may therefore render search for *T. pallidum* by dark-field microscopy useless.

d. T

e. F—After even one dose of penicillin, *T. pallidum* will no longer be detectable in the lesion.

A.14.2 a. T

b. T

c. T

d. T

e. T

A.14.3 a. T—This is a very sensitive test of neurosyphilis in the CSF although it yields false positives in some normal patients.

b. T—This is the basic pathological defect in GPI which leads to:

c. T—Secondary cerebral atrophy.

d. T—This is the clinical result of cerebral atrophy.

e. F—These are rarely found in GPI.

A.14.4 a. T—This is one of the commonest features of secondary syphilis.

b. T—Uveitis, both symptomatic and silent, are found in early syphilis.

c. F

d. F—This is a feature of tertiary syphilis.

e. F—The "sign of the groove" is a description of inguinal lymphadenopathy both above and below the inguinal ligament, with the "groove" being the ligament itself. It is usually associated with lymphogranuloma venereum.

Q.14.5 The following are true of early syphilis:

a. Up to 40% of patients' CSF contain *T. pallidum* prior to treatment
b. Early syphilitic hepatitis is unusual in that the alkaline phosphatase is disproportionately raised (i.e. it appears to be an obstructive hepatitis)
c. Uveitis never occurs
d. Aortic regurgitation is a known manifestation of this stage of syphilis
e. At this stage of the disease the causative organism is disseminated around the body

Q.14.6 In untreated acquired syphilis:

a. Cardiovascular complications probably occur in 10% of cases
b. Neurosyphilis occurs in 20% of cases
c. Gummata occur in 10% of cases
d. Stigma of late disease may develop within 10 years of the primary infection
e. Hutchinson's triad occurs in 15% of cases

Q.14.7 In primary syphilis:

a. All the serological tests are usually positive early on
b. The serological tests usually become positive in the sequence FTA, *Treponema pallidum* haemagglutination test (TPHA), Venereal Disease Research Laboratory Test (VDRL)
c. The serological tests usually become positive in the sequence FTA, VDRL, TPHA
d. The FTA is only positive late in primary syphilis
e. If treated early enough, all the serological tests may revert to negative

For answers see page 134

A Syphilitic Story

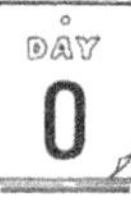

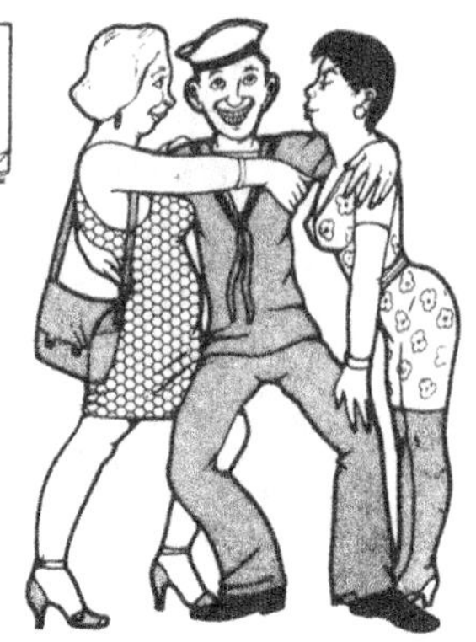

Three weeks ago the ship dropped anchor.

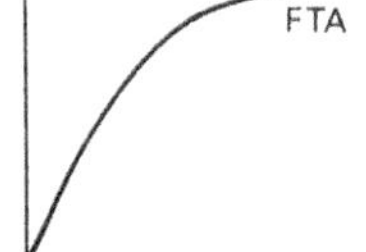

Now sailor John has a penile chancre,
He wished from the girls he stayed away,
'Cause now he got an FTA.

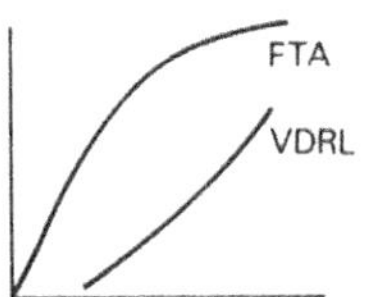

"You might have syph", the docs foretell,
Day 28 shows VDRL.

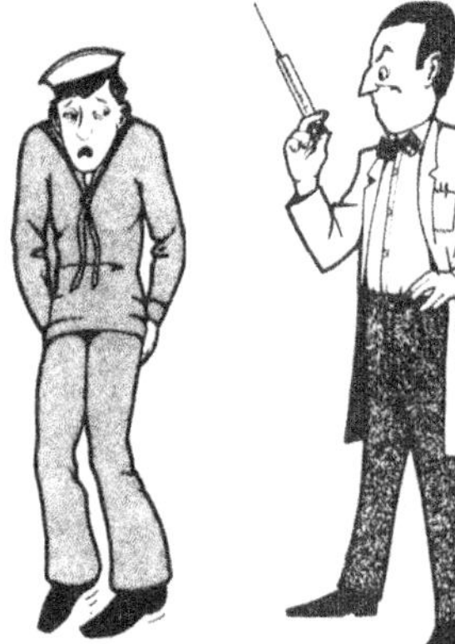

"The needle you need with penicillin",
The doctors say with sardonic grinning,
"Oh no!", says John "I'll not have
Penicillin in a jab."

DAY
42

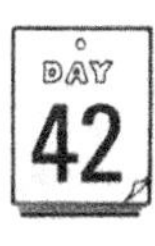

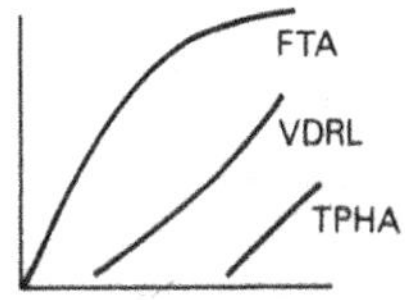

So off he goes, 2 weeks away
And returns to docs with TPHA.

DAY
70
FTA pos.
TPHA pos
VDRL 1:64

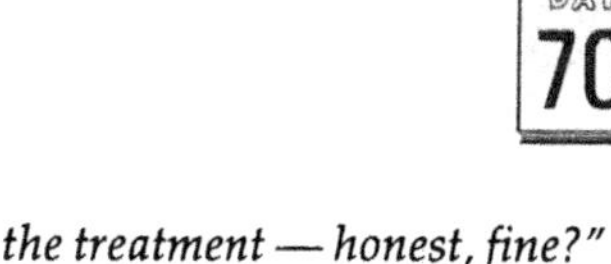

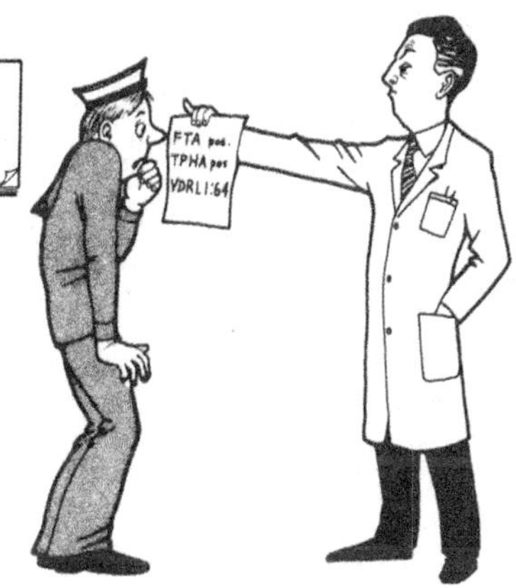

"I'll take the treatment — honest, fine?"
But only returns in 4 weeks' time
He blinds his sorrows with some hash,
And disregards his macular rash.

"Please come back" the docs implore,
"Your VDRL's 1:64."

YEAR
1

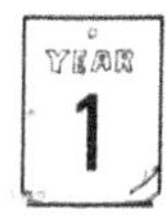

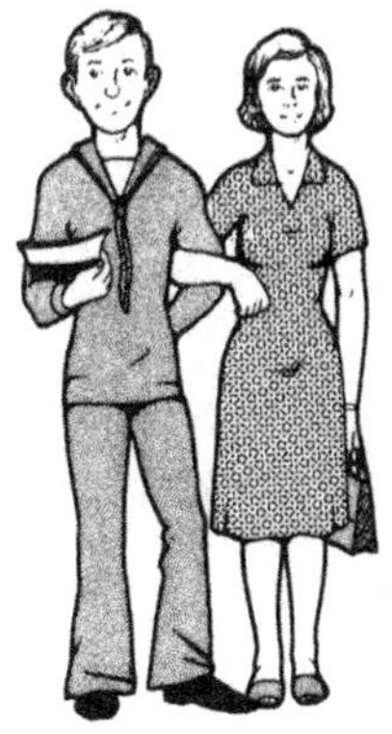

He takes the treatment, it's not so bad,
The macules go, he's really glad.

A year has gone, he's a changed man,
He's going steady with his Jan,
The VDRL has gone away,
Not so the serum TPHA,
Which like the positive FTA,
Will stay with him till dying day.

If only he'd been treated fast,
None of the tests would stay to last.

Answers

A.14.5 a. T

b. T

c. F—Uveitis is rarely symptomatic but more commonly clinically silent at this stage.

d. F—This is a manifestation of tertiary syphilis.

e. T

A.14.6 a. T

b. F—Neurosyphilis occurs in 10% of cases.

c. F—Gummata occur in 15% of cases. No stigma of late disease is reported in 65% of untreated cases.

d. T

e. F—Hutchinson's triad (interstitial keratitis, Hutchinson's teeth and eight nerve deafness) is a late feature of congenital syphilis.

A.14.7 a. F

b. F

c. T

d. T

e. T

Q.14.8 The treatment of choice in syphilis is:

a. Metronidazole
b. Tetracycline
c. Penicillin
d. Erythromycin
e. Cotrimoxazole

Q.14.9 The following conditions are associated with chronic biological false-positive reactions in the non-specific (reagin) serological tests (e.g. the VDRL):

a. Pregnancy
b. Sarcoidosis
c. Herpes simplex infection
d. Systemic lupus erythematosis
e. Intravenous drug abuse

Q.14.10 In secondary syphilis:

a. All the serological tests for syphilis are positive
b. The VDRL reagin titre is usually high
c. The VDRL titre is usually negative
d. The FTA and TPHA may be negative
e. The prozone phenomenon can occur

For answers see over

A.14.8 a. F—Metronidazole is used in the therapy of *Trichomonas vaginalis* and bacterial vaginosis. It has a minor treponemicidal effect.
b. F—Tetracycline is the first-line alternative to penicillin in patients allergic to this drug.
c. T
d. F—Erythromycin is the second-line alternative in treatment. It is safe to use in pregnancy but has poor placental transfer. The infant should be retreated at birth with penicillin.
e. F—Cotrimoxazole has no action on *T. pallidum*. It may be prescribed whilst investigating patients for syphilis.

A.14.9 a. F—Pregnancy is associated with an acute biological false-positive reaction in the non-specific serology test. This occurs in 5% of normal pregnancies and reverts to normal within 6 months.
b. T—Granulomatous conditions (e.g. leprosy, tuberculosis and sarcoidosis) are associated with a chronic biological false-positive reaction which is present for greater than 6 months.
c. F—Viral infections (e.g. herpes simplex) are associated with an acute biological false-positive reaction.
d. T—Autoimmune disorders (e.g. systemic lupus erythematosus) are associated with chronic biological false-positive reaction.
e. T

A.14.10 a. T
b. T
c. F
d. F
e. T—Where there is an excess of reagin antibody the test may appear negative unless the serum is diluted.

Q.14.11 The following features are well recognised features of tabes dorsalis:

a. "Lightening" pains in the legs, occurring at right angles to the length of the long bone
b. Absent triceps jerks
c. Dulled ankle jerks
d. Brisk ankle jerks
e. Ataxia worse in the dark

Q.14.12 A 42-year-old homosexual man comes to the clinic for a check. No penile, anal or oral lesions are seen. Syphilis serology is as follows:

FTA antibody negative, TPHA negative, VDRL 1:16. Such a clinical picture is likely to be due to:

a. A rectal chancre
b. Systemic lupus erythematosus
c. A cerebral glioma
d. A recent vaccination
e. Tuberculosis of the chest

Q.14.13 The following is (are) true of syphilitic aortic regurgitation:

a. It may coexist with angina due to coronary ostial stenosis
b. Systemic steroids should be given prior to antisyphilitic treatment to prevent coronary ostial occlusion as a consequence of treatment
c. There may be coexistent brachial artery inequality (in pulse and blood pressure)
d. It usually coexists with an aortic abdominal aneurysm
e. It may coexist with Argyll–Robertson pupils

Q.14.14 Benzathine penicillin, 2.4 × 10^6 units i.m., is adequate treatment for:

a. Neurosyphilis
b. Late latent syphilis
c. Secondary syphilis
d. Primary syphilis
e. Early latent syphilis

For answers see over

A.14.11 a. T—These are very painful but short lived.
b. F—The upper limbs are not commonly affected in tabes.
c. T
d. F
e. T—The posteror column disease leads to ataxia that is compensated by vision so that in the dark the ataxia becomes exaggerated.

A.14.12 a. F—A rectal chancre (primary syphilis) would probably have converted the serology to positive throughout if the VDRL is 1:16. Very rarely this serological picture might be seen in primary syphilis.
b. T—The serology suggests a biologically false positive (BFP) reaction to reagin (VDRL).
c. F—This is not a cause of a BFP.
d. T—This is a cause of an acute BFP reaction.
e. T—See b) above.

A.14.13 a. T—Aortic aneurysm (classically the ascending thoracic aorta) is a manifestation of tertiary syphilis. This may result in coronary ostial stenosis due to syphilitic endarteritis.
b. T—Steroids are said to prevent the Jarisch-Herxheimer reaction, which causes oedema.
c. T—The aortic endarteritis may cause inequalities in the blood flow of the brachial artery roots.
d. F—Classically syphilitic aneurysms affect the thoracic (ascending) aorta only.
e. T—Tabes dorsalis and aortic aneurysm may coexist.

A.14.14 a. F
b. F
c. T
d. T
e. T

The above treatment is adequate for any stage up to early latent syphilis. It gives a continuous serum level of greater than the treponemocidal level of penicillin (>0.018 mg/litre) for just over a week.

Q.14.15 A mother's serological tests for syphilis are:

FTA positive, TPHA positive, VDRL positive 1:2.

Congenital syphilis in her newborn child is strongly suggested by:

a. Finding *T. pallidum* in moist skin lesions on the baby
b. Finding the neonatal serum VDRL titre is positive with undiluted serum
c. Finding the neonatal FTA antibody IgM is positive
d. Finding the neonatal FTA antibody IgG is positive
e. Knowing the mother has received cotrimoxazole for 2 weeks in the recent past

A tertiary syphilitic can crawl,
In darkness but not walk at all,
His posterior columns,
Are down in the doldrums,
And so make him stumble and fall.

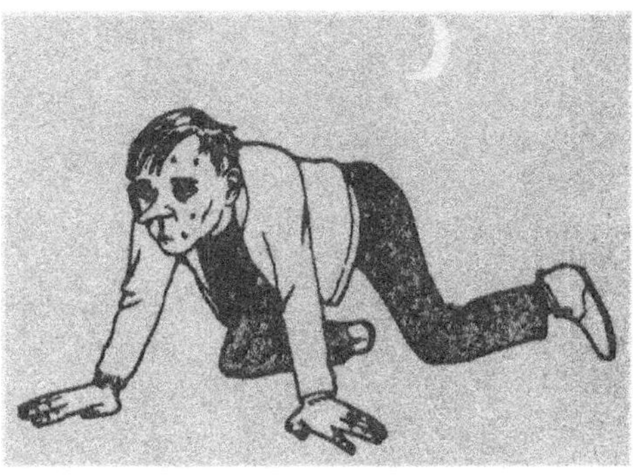

Tabes dorsalis in a manifestation of tertiary syphilis. Degeneration of the spinal posterior columns leads to ataxia and a high stepping gait. This becomes decompensated if the visual input is removed, e.g. at night. Nowadays in the United Kingdom diabetic (mellitus) pseudo tabes is a commoner cause than syphilis of this problem.

For answers see over

A.14.15 a. T—These confirm the presence of early congenital syphilis.
b. F—If the neonatal VDRL titre is much higher than the maternal titre, the implication is that there is an active infection in the child.
c. T—FTA IgG may be passively transferred from the maternal circulation. IgM is too large to pass the fetomaternal barrier, so that it indicates active infection in the child.
d. F—See c) above.
e. F—Cotrimoxazole will have no effect on the infection.

Q.14.16 Hutchinson's triad for congenital syphilis is:

a. Moon's molars
b. Notched incisor teeth
c. Interstitial keratitis
d. Chorioretinitis
e. Eighth cranial nerve deafness

Q.14.17 The aetiological agent of syphilis is:

a. *Treponema pertenue*
b. *Treponema pallidum*
c. *Treponema carateum*
d. *Treponema macrodentium*
e. *Treponema microdentium*

Q.14.18 Argyll–Robertson pupils:

a. Are usually found in patients with late congenital neurosyphilis
b. Are pupils that are pinpoint in size, react to accommodation but not to light
c. Are the same as syphilitic pupils
d. May be the result of diabetes mellitus
e. May rarely occur in primary syphilis

Q.14.19 The following regimes consistently result in treponemacidal levels of antibiotic in the CSF:

a. Benzathine penicillin 2.4 mu weekly for 4 weeks
b. Intravenous penicillin G (4×10^6 units and probenecid 6 hourly)
c. Procaine penicillin 2.4×10^6 i.m. units daily and probenecid 6 hourly
d. Amoxicillin 2.0 g thrice daily plus probenecid twice daily
e. Penicillin V 1000 mg and probenecid 6 hourly

For answers see over

A.14.16 a. F
b. T
c. T
d. F
e. T

All of the above are found in congenital syphilis whether early or late. The true answers were, however, described by Hutchinson.

A.14.17 a. F—*Treponema pertenue* is the aetiological agent in Yaws.
b. T—*Treponema pallidum* is the aetiological agent in venereal and endemic syphilis.
c. F—*Treponema carateum* is the aetiological agent in pinta.
d. F—*Treponema macrodentium* is a saprophytic treponeme of the mouth.
e. F—*Treponema microdentium* is a saprophytic treponeme of the mouth.

A.14.18 a. F
b. T—However, sluggishly reactive pupils (to light) found in the presence of tabes dorsalis strongly suggest tertiary syphilis. They are not Argyll–Robertson pupils but are "syphilitic" pupils.
c. F—See b) above.
d. T—Diabetic pseudotabes causes Argyll–Robertson pupils.
e. F

A.14.19 a. F
b. T
c. T
d. T
e. F

There are strong theoretical arguments for using one of treatments b), c) or d) for patients with neurosyphilis.

Q.14.20 Typical characteristics of the primary sore or chancre of syphilis are:

a. Painful
b. Painless
c. Usually single
d. Usually multiple
e. Usually associated with enlarged, firm rubbery local lymphadenopathy

Q.14.21 The following clinical pictures are found in acquired tertiary syphilis:

a. Mid-diastolic heart murmur
b. Hutchinson's incisors
c. Bony gummata
d. Clinical depression
e. Corrigan pulse

Q.14.22 The first serological test for syphilis to become positive in primary syphilis is usually:

a. The TPHA
b. The FTA
c. The VDRL
d. The Wassermann reaction
e. The *T. pallidum* complement fixation test

For answers see over

A.14.20 a. F—The primary chancre is characteristically painless.
b. T
c. T
d. F—The primary chancre is characteristically single.
e. T—The lymphadenopathy at the site of the drainage of the primary site is characteristically unilateral and painless.

A.14.21 a. F—Syphilitic aortic regurgitation causes an early diagnostic murmur.
b. F—Hutchinson's incisors are one of the three "stigmata" of congenital syphilis.
c. T—These are the commonest manifestations of untreated tertiary syphilis.
d. T—Clinical depression is found in early GPI.
e. T—This is found in aortic regurgitation.

A.14.22 a. F
b. T
c. F
d. F
e. F

Q.14.23 A patient has the following serological tests for treponemal disease: TPHA positive, FTA antibody positive, VDRL negative.

They are consistent with:

a. Untreated Yaws (25 years ago)
b. Late latent syphilis
c. Secondary syphilis
d. Primary syphilis
e. Tabes dorsalis

Q.14.24 Features of secondary syphilis include:

a. An itchy generalised rash
b. Generalised lymphadenopathy
c. Snail-track ulcers
d. Condyloma acuminata
e. Alopecia areata

Q.14.25 The following should be considered in the differential diagnosis of a primary chancre:

a. Chancroid
b. Lymphogranuloma venereum
c. Genital herpes simplex virus infection
d. Anal fissure
e. Pilonidal sinus

For answers see over

A.14.23 a. T—Syphilis or yaws acquired some years previously, whether treated or untreated, are consistent with this serology pattern.
b. T—See a) above.
c. F—If a prozone (antibody in great excess causing a negative) is not checked for, the VDRL will be apparently negative until the serum is diluted. There is a high VDRL titre in secondary syphilis.
d. T—In primary syphilis the VDRL usually, but not always, reverts to positive after the FTA antibody but before the TPHA.
e. T—The VDRL titre in tabes dorsalis may be raised but not uncommonly is negative.

A.14.24 a. F—Classically, a non-itchy generalised rash ranging from macular to papulosquamous in character, and affecting all sites including the palms and soles, is found.
b. T
c. T—Mucous membrane lesions are highly infectious.
d. F—Condyloma acuminata or genital warts should not be confused with the condyloma lata of secondary syphilis.
e. F—Alopecia areata is an autoimmune disorder characterised by exclamation mark hairs.

A.14.25 a. T—These conditions are all considered in the differential diagnosis of genital ulcer disease and primary syphilis.
b. T—See a) above.
c. T—See a) above.
d. T—See a) above.
e. F

15. *Miscellaneous*

Q.15.1 Drugs that may be safely given in the first trimester of pregnancy include:

a. Ampicillin
b. Metronidazole
c. Acyclovir
d. Tetracycline
e. Erythromycin

Q.15.2 The following are well-recognised adverse reactions:

a. Vomiting following acyclovir administration
b. A fixed-drug eruption following tetracycline administration
c. Nausea, vomiting and/or diarrhoea in patients taking erythromycin
d. The Jarisch–Herxheimer (JH) reaction after injection with spectinomycin
e. Thinning of the skin after application of clotrimazole cream

Q.15.3 Drug interactions:

a. Food, especially dairy products, causes decreased absorption of tetracycline by 50% or more
b. Iron-supplementing drugs should be taken at least 2 h apart from tetracyclines
c. Patients using oral contraceptives should discontinue the pill when taking antibiotics because of drug interaction
d. Sulphonamides may be given to patients on warfarin without adjustment of warfarin dosage
e. Patients who imbibe alcohol while taking metronidazole may experience palpitations, tachycardia, flushing and nausea

For answers see over

Answers

A.15.1 a. T
b. F
c. F
d. F
e. T

Metronidazole has theoretical objections but these are not confirmed by clinical trials. Acyclovir has not been tested and tetracycline is not given due to its effect on the fetal teeth and bones although this effect occurs in late pregnancy.

Ampicillin and erythromycin have been used in early pregnancy with no ill effects.

A.15.2 a. F—Remarkably few side effects have been observed with acyclovir (renal toxicity in dehydrated patients is one).
b. T—Ulceration occurs, often around the coronal sulcus. May become secondarily infected.
c. T
d. F—The JH reaction occurs after commencing treatment for early syphilis and causes fever and flu-like effects. Spectinomycin cannot be used to treat syphilis.
e. F—Occurs with strong steroid-containing creams and not with clotrimazole.

A.15.3 a. T
b. T—Iron chelates tetracyclines and, therefore, they should not coexist in the stomach.
c. F—Interaction may occur, e.g. with ampicillin, and is often idiosyncratic. Patients should continue oral contraception but should always be warned about the possibility of reduced contraceptive efficacy.
d. F—Sulphonamides displace warfarin from protein-binding sites and enhance hypoprothrombinaemia — therefore dosage adjustment is required.
e. T—Disulfiram reaction. Apparently due to inhibition of metabolism of ethanol and acetaldehyde by metronidazole.

Q.15.4 The following is true of acute anaphylaxis after penicillin (ampicillin) treatment:

a. The most important therapeutic action is to give 100 mg i.v. hydrocortisone as a bolus
b. The most important therapeutic action is to give 5 ml 1:10 000 adrenaline intramuscularly into the pectoral muscles
c. It may follow oral amoxycillin
d. It may present with the patient feeling they have been killed by the doctor or nurse who gave the injection of procaine penicillin
e. It may lead to bronchospasm

Q.15.5 An 18-year-old sexually active homosexual heroin addict tells you he had shared needles in the past. Although a manual worker, he has three splinter haemorrhages in his fingernails. He is well, but is known to carry hepatitis B surface antigen and HIV antibody. He has had severe toothache plus jaw swelling for 3 days and tells you that throughout his life he has been allergic to a large amount of fish. He has immune complexes to IgM detectable in serum.

Which of the following could cause the immune complexes:

a. SBE (subacute bacterial endocarditis)
b. Tooth (root) abscess (e.g. staphylococci)
c. Fish allergy
d. Hepatitis B
e. HIV

Q.15.6 The following are true of perihepatitis:

a. It may be caused by *Treponema pallidum*
b. It may be caused by *Neisseria gonorrhoeae*
c. It may be caused by *Chlamydia trachomatis*
d. Clinically it is always associated with pelvic pain
e. Liver function tests are often normal

For answers see over

A.15.4 a. F—The most important first move is to give adrenaline. This may be life saving. Antihistamine and steroids may be given after this.
b. T—See a) above.
c. T—Acute anaphylaxis has been reported to occur within ½ h of oral ingestion of amoxycillin.
d. F—This is the procaine reaction — not anaphylaxis.
e. T

A.15.5 a. T
b. T
c. T
d. T
e. T

All of the above antigens may result in the formation of the immune complexes.

A.15.6 a. F—Syphilis can cause a *hepatitis* in the secondary stage and intrahepatic gummata in the tertiary stage but not perihepatitis (inflammation of the liver capsule).
b. T—These organisms are thought to infect the liver capsule via genital tract infections.
c. T—See b) above.
d. F—It is not always associated with pelvic pain.
e. T—Liver function tests are usually normal, as the liver itself is not directly involved in the pathology. However, one or other of the parameters of LFTs may be slightly raised, e.g. bilirubin.

Q.15.7 Urethral syndrome:

a. Is defined as dysuria and frequency in the absence of bladder bacteruria ($<10^5$ organisms/ml urine)
b. Is defined as dysuria and frequency in the presence of bladder bacteruria ($>10^5$ organisms/ml urine)
c. Is always associated with underlying renal pathology
d. May be associated with the symptoms of haematuria and loin pain
e. Is also called abacterial cystitis

Q.15.8 Ureaplasma urealyticum:

a. Is a urea-splitting mycoplasma
b. Is commonly found in the male urethra without evidence of urethritis
c. Strains have been inoculated intraurethrally into human volunteers
d. Microorganisms are resistant to tetracyclines in about 10% of clinical isolates
e. Is an important cause of epididymitis

For answers see over

A.15.7 a. T
b. F
c. F—The urethral syndrome is not associated with renal pathology.
d. T
e. T—But conventionally there may be bacteria present but not at a concentration of $>10^5$ organisms/ml.

A.15.8 a. T
b. T—The presence of ureaplasmas in the genital tract of men and women is directly related to the number of sexual partners they have had: it is therefore an index of promiscuity. However, in certain circumstances, it may be pathogenic.
c. T—At least three male human volunteers have had ureaplasmas inoculated intraurethrally and all developed urethritis. Despite treatment with tetracycline, one individual had persistent urinary threads for 6 months, suggesting that ureaplasmas could initiate chronic disease.
d. T—Tetracycline-resistant ureaplasmas may be responsible for some cases of persistent NGU. The organisms will respond to treatment with erythromycin.
e. F

Ureaplasma urealyticum
Is found in the urethras of some
Famous medical men,
And we have it from them
T'was instilled by pipette and not fun.

Q.15.9 The following epidemiological statements are true about England and Wales in the mid-1980s:

a. Syphilis is slightly increasing in incidence
b. Genital herpes simplex is being increasingly reported
c. Wart virus infection (HPV) of the genitalia is static in incidence
d. Non-specific genital infection is on the increase
e. The total number of patients attending VD clinics is increasing annually

Q.15.10 Meningitis:

a. May be the result of infection with *N. gonorrhoeae*
b. Is a common finding in patients with primary genital herpes
c. When associated with a purpuric rash, is usually due to *N. gonorrhoeae*
d. May present insidiously when caused by *Cryptosporidium*
e. Is always caused by syphilis when the CSF FTA is positive

Q.15.11 The differential diagnosis of orogenital blisters in an adult should include:

a. Chicken pox
b. Measles
c. Syphilis
d. Drug allergies
e. Herpes zoster (shingles)

Q.15.12 Which of the following should be considered as a possible differential diagnosis in a 58-year-old man with a penile ulcer:

a. Primary syphilis
b. Behcet's disease
c. Plasma cell balanitis of Zoon
d. Squamous cell carcinoma
e. Genital warts that have been treated too vigorously

For answers see over

A.15.9 a. F—Syphilis rates have markedly decreased since the Second World War and have remained relatively static at a low level since the 1960s.

b. T—This may be due to an actual increase in prevalence of the disease and/or because of greater awareness of the condition and a higher level of reporting the condition.

c. F—There has been a gradual increase in the rates of genital HPV in the last 10 years.

d. T

e. T

A.15.10 a. T—Gonococcal meningitis is very rare.

b. F—Herpes simplex meningitis consequent on primary genital herpes is rare. Meningism is commoner.

c. F—The neisserial infection associated with purpura is meningococcal.

d. F—*Cryptosporidium* causes watery diarrhoea. *Cryptococcus* causes subacute meningitis.

e. F—An isolated FTA in the CSF when all other parameters are negative may be a false-positive result. The FTA is a very sensitive, perhaps an oversensitive, test that need not necessarily indicate the presence of neurosyphilis. If other CSF parameters are positive, e.g. an excess of white cells, the patient almost certainly has neurosyphilis.

A.15.11 a. T

b. F—Does not cause vesiculation.

c. F—Does not cause vesiculation.

d. T

e. F—Shingles would not occur in the oral and genital areas simultaneously.

A.15.12 a. T—Primary syphilis causes a painless ulcer.

b. T—Behcet's disease causes painful genital ulceration on the penis and/or scrotum.

c. F—This does not generally cause ulceration.

d. T

e. T—Excessive treatment of warts may lead to iatrogenic ulceration.

Q.15.13 Painful inguinal lymphadenopathy:

a. May be found in genital herpes simplex infection
b. Is found in infection with some strains of *Chlamydia trachomatis*
c. Is common in primary syphilis
d. Is a feature of granuloma inguinale
e. Is found in patients with chancroid

Q.15.14 Genital ulcers:

a. In industrialised Western countries are more common than urethritis or vaginitis
b. Are usually caused by herpes simplex virus infection in Western countries
c. May be caused by syphilitic infection
d. Are often the result of chancroid in Asia and Africa
e. May be caused by drug therapy

Q.15.15 Penicillin:

a. Is the only effective treatment for syphilis
b. Is effective treatment for non-gonococcal urethritis
c. Is ineffective against β-lactamase-producing strains of gonorrhoea
d. Must be given daily to treat uncomplicated syphilis successfully
e. Is a useful drug to use for pelvic inflammatory disease of uncertain aetiology

For answers see over

A.15.13 a. T
b. T—Lymphogranuloma venereum strains of *C. trachomatis* cause grossly enlarged tender inguinal adenopathy.
c. F—Primary syphilis characteristically leads to unilateral painless lymphadenopathy.
d. F—Granuloma inguinale does not result in lymphadenopathy.
e. T

A.15.14 a. F
b. T
c. T
d. T
e. T

A.15.15 a. F—Tetracycline, doxycycline, cefuroxime and, to a lesser extent, erythromycin are also effective.
b. F—Ineffective: not antichlamydial.
c. T—Penicillin is destroyed by these organisms by enzyme action.
d. F—Various long-acting regimes, e.g. benzathine penicillin may be given weekly. However, this regime is apparently unable to eradicate the organism from the CSF and may be inadequate in neurosyphilis.
e. F—Not useful because it is inactive against *C. trachomatis* and has limited activity against Gram-negative organisms.

Q.15.16 Pubic lice:

a. Commonly infest sexually active people aged 15–25 years
b. Are the same lice as infest the head and body
c. Cannot be seen with the naked eye
d. Lay eggs which hatch within 9 days
e. Are vectors for relapsing fever

Q.15.17 When treating scabies:

a. Only areas with obvious lesions require the topical application of gamma benzene hexachloride
b. There is absolutely no risk in pregnancy
c. There is rapid relief of symptoms within 24 h of therapy
d. All members of the household and sexual contacts should be treated
e. Irritant contact dermatitis is not uncommon

Q.15.18 The lesions in scabies:

a. Characteristically are non-irritant
b. Characteristically occur on the hands, wrists, elbows and face
c. May exhibit burrows
d. Are usually polymorphous
e. May resemble those of secondary syphilis

For answers see over

A.15.16 a. T—The commonest mode of transmission is direct skin contact. Therefore, it occurs in the most sexually active.
b. F—There are three types of louse: head, body, pubic.
c. F—Nits are at least 0.8 × 0.3 mm and the louse is larger.
d. T
e. F—The vector for relapsing fever is the body louse.

A.15.17 a. F—The entire skin surface below the head should be treated to ensure eradication of all mites.
b. F—There is insufficient toxicological data to support this claim and, therefore, caution is advisable in treating patients.
c. F—Infectivity ceases after 24 h but symptoms may persist for several weeks.
d. T—It may take 2 months from contact until development of symptoms and, therefore, even asymptomatic contacts require treatment.
e. T—Usually from overuse of therapy.

A.15.18 a. F—Lesions are itchy, especially at night.
b. F—The lesions of scabies characteristically occur in the webs of fingers, the palmar surface of the wrists, anterior shoulders, buttocks and genitalia.
c. T
d. T
e. T—Secondary syphilis and scabies may both exhibit a papular rash. The latter, unlike the former, is itchy.

Q.15.19 A Bartholin's abscess:

a. Is usually unilateral
b. Is always associated with sexually transmitted disease
c. May be prevented by salt baths
d. The treatment includes drainage and suture of the cyst wall to the surrounding skin.
e. May recur even after surgical treatment

Q.15.20 Vulval dystrophy:

a. May present with pruritus
b. Is only found in postmenopausal women
c. Is associated with white patches on the vulval skin
d. Is always premalignant
e. Can be categorised by careful history and examination

For answers see over

A.15.19 a. T
b. F
c. F
d. T
e. T

Although *Chlamydia trachomatis* and the gonococcus have been associated with abscesses, this is not invariably so. Salt baths have no effect. Although a recent study showed encouraging results for treatment by needle aspiration and antibiotic therapy, most cases are treated by the method described as marsupialisation. Although this procedure is designed to prevent recurrence, it is still possible for the problem to recur.

A.15.20 a. T
b. F
c. T
d. F
e. F

Pruritus may be the only presenting complaint. Although more common after the menopause, it may occur in younger women. It is not invariably premalignant, although some types are so. Colposcopy may aid diagnosis and allow accurate biopsy of individual lesions for histological diagnosis. An increasing number of cases of premalignant disease known as vulval intraepithelial neoplasia (VIN) are being satisfactorily treated by local laser vaporisation.

16. *Case Histories*

Q.16.1 Mandy, a 17-year-old girl, has had recurrent *Trichomonas vaginalis* for 6 weeks.

In fact, on closer inspection of her case, you find that in spite of conventional courses of oral metronidazole (2.0 g as a loading dose, and 400 mg bd for 5 days) she has never eliminated this organism during the 6 weeks.

The following are appropriate ways of managing her case:

a. Estimate the metronidazole levels in the blood after oral ingestion.
b. Take a bacterial culture of a high vaginal swab and see if any other vaginal organisms metabolise metronidazole.
c. Do in vitro sensitivity of the *T. vaginalis* to metronidazole.
d. Try giving metronidazole 800 mg tds for a week in the hope that it will work.
e. Treat the male partner for *T. vaginalis*.

Q.16.2 A 40-year-old actor, Timothy, complains to you he is losing his memory. He has become morose, anxious and clinically depressed. He is known to be HIV antibody positive. On direct questioning he tells you he has smoked 60 cigarettes a day for 25 years.

Clinically there are signs of short-term memory loss, nominal asphasia and impaired two-point discrimination.

His serological tests for syphilis are as follows:
TPHA positive, VDRL negative, FTA positive.

Which of the following are a possible diagnosis:

a. Carcinoma of the bronchus with cerebral secondaries
b. General paresis of the insane (GPI)
c. Psychotic depression
d. HIV disease of the brain
e. Cryptococcal meningitis

For answers see over

Answers

A.16.1 a. T—If this is below the level suggested by the in vitro sensitivity test, there may be problems with absorption.
b. T—Some vaginal bacteria, e.g. streptococci, may metabolise metronidazole, thus decreasing the amount available to act on *T. vaginalis*.
c. T—To screen for in vitro resistance.
d. T—Sometimes large doses seem successfully to eradicate the organism.
e. T

A.16.2 a. T
b. T—The syphilis serology and clinical state are consistent with a diagnosis of GPI.
c. F—Psychotic depression would not lead to such specific clinical signs as are described here but might globally impair concentration, memory and perception.
d. T—HIV disease can cause a dementing process.
e. T—Cryptococcal meningitis causes malaise, fever and symptoms and signs of meningitis and if left untreated may lead to signs of encephalitis.

Q.16.3 Steven, an 18-year-old medical student, comes to a clinic for screening tests to exclude sexually transmitted disease.

He has had intercourse with four casual female contacts in the last month, but has no symptoms. He is uncircumcised. He last passed urine 2 h previously. A urethral smear shows five pus cells per high-power field and numerous secondary organisms (skin flora). A monoclonal slide for *Chlamydia trachomatis* is negative; first-catch urine looks clear.

Which of the following statements are true:

a. He has low-grade non-gonococcal urethritis (NGU)
b. His tests are normal
c. His tests indicate a low-grade balanitis rather than urethritis
d. Tests should be repeated on him, with him holding his urine for at least 4 h
e. Tests should be repeated on him but with the glans cleansed with normal saline before milking the urethra to test for urethritis

For answers see over

A.16.3 a. F
b. F
c. T
d. T
e. T

Although the minimum number of pus cells per high-power field in order to diagnose urethritis is five cells per high-power field, this presumes that there are no secondary organisms present. If they are present, with a low pus cell count (i.e. five) and no threads in the first-catch urine, a low-grade balanitis is being sampled, resulting in the above results.

Steps d) and e) should be taken to screen for urethritis rather than low-grade balanitis.

Q.16.4 Peter, a 29-year-old asthmatic homosexual, has been a nervous person all his life. When he found out he was HIV antibody positive a year ago, he took up smoking, so that now he gets through a packet of 20 cigarettes a day. Three months before his current visit, he was admitted to the wards, when hysterical hyperventilation was diagnosed. He now tells you that he gets attacks of shortness of breath at exercise and at rest. Finally, in tears, he tells you that a private doctor put him on diazepam 8 weeks ago, but that he came off this last week. Clinical examination of the chest is unremarkable, except for a few expiratory rhonci heard all over the chest.

How would you manage him initially?

a. Tell him he was suffering from panic attacks on withdrawing from diazepam and reassure him
b. Renew his prescription for salbutamol inhaler and review his progress as an outpatient
c. Arrange a bronchoscopy and lung biopsy to confirm the diagnosis
d. Put him on a high dose of cotrimoxazole because the most likely diagnosis is *Pneumocytis carinii* pneumonia
e. Do white cell subsets on him to assess his level of immunodeficiency
f. Do a chest X-ray, his blood gases and lung function and assess his progress as an inpatient

For answers see over

A.16.4 a. F—This may be true, but unless further investigated immediately he may die of other more serious illnesses.

b. F—Asthma may be the cause of his symptoms but he should be observed in the wards to make the correct diagnosis.

c. F—This investigation has a definite morbidity and mortality even in expert hands; less-invasive initial tests should precede it. He may have hysterical hyperventilation again — see f).

d. F—*Pneumocytis carinii* pneumonia (PCP) may be the diagnosis. However, diagnosis before treatment is mandatory in this patient as there are a number of possibilities.

e. F—The best assessment of his immunological status is his clinical state, i.e. has he PCP or not?

f. T—Proceed according to the results. He may need bronchoscopy.

Q.16.5 A 32-year-old homosexual man had one episode of active anal intercourse with another man who had hepatitis B and AIDS. You see him 4 months after this episode. He tells you he had a severe febrile illness lasting 'weeks' some weeks ago but is now much better. He is worried about which infection he picked up. Another hospital told him a week before he sees you that he was HIV antibody, hepatitis B surface antigen and antibody negative and that his liver function tests were normal. He has never received a hepatitis B vaccine and was told he was 'not immune to hepatitis B' 6 months ago.

Which of the following actions are correct:

a. Tell him he has not acquired hepatitis B
b. Tell him he may have acquired HIV infection and that he should be retested in 6 months
c. Tell him he may have acquired hepatitis B and look for hepatitis B core antibody
d. Tell him he is more likely to acquire hepatitis B than HIV disease from this one episode of intercourse
e. Ask him if he had enlarged lymph nodes at the time of the acute illness

Q.16.6 A 45-year-old businessman travels to India and South Africa over a 3-week period during which he has intercourse with prostitutes. He took one tetracycline (500-mg) tablet after seeing the last girl and 24 h later develops a penile ulcer. It is a little tender, smelly and somewhat indurated. The inguinal area is 'fuller' than you expect but there are no obvious glands.

What investigations would you order?

a. Syphilis serology with FTA
b. *Chlamydia trachomatis* culture of the ulcer
c. Herpes simplex culture of ulcer material
d. Smears of granuloma inguinale from the ulcer
e. Smears and cultures to exclude chancroid
f. Re-exposure to tetracycline under controlled conditions

For answers see over

A.16.5 a. F—This cannot be stated categorically on the above data—see c).

b. T—Not all patients become HIV antibody positive even some weeks after they have the viraemia.

c. T—After acute hepatitis B before surface antibody has formed, the only evidence for this infection may be the core antibody (IgM and IgG). This is called the 'window period'.

d. T—Hepatitis B is more infectious that HIV infection.

e. T—This would favour acute HIV disease rather than hepatitis B.

A.16.6 a. T—In spite of taking a tetracycline tablet, he still may be developing syphilis. The earliest serological test to become positive would be the FTA.

b. T—This lesion could be lymphogranuloma venereum although absence of lymphadenopathy and the conspicuous penile lesion are against this diagnosis.

c. T—This is a very likely pathogen here.

d. T—Granuloma inguinale may cause exhuberant 'ulcers' with no lymphadenopathy.

e. T

f. F—Fixed drug eruption to tetracycline is possible, but re-exposure to this would certainly make the lesions worse.

Q.16.7 A 37-year-old man had his first attack of non-gonococcal urethritis 6 months before he sees you. He complains that in spite of a course of doxycycline and erythromycin, he still has premicturition urethral discharge which he can milk out of the urethra most mornings.

A recent MSU showed a moderate sterile pyuria but two previous such specimens were normal. He has a past history of gonococcal urethritis which remained untreated for 3 weeks while he was working as a mercenary in Africa. His current girlfriend has also received recent courses of doxycycline and erythromycin.

Which course of action is appropriate?

a. A first-catch urine that shows 'threads' should be followed by a 2-week course of tetracycline in the first place
b. He should be screened for prostatitis by looking at expressed prostatic fluid
c. He should have an intravenous urethrogram and ascending urethrography
d. His urethral meatus should be everted to inspect the urethral mucosa
e. He should be treated for *Trichomonas vaginalis*
f. Tell him to squeeze out the urethral discharge each morning so as to prevent blockage of the paraurethral glands
g. Order 'Stamey tests', i.e. bacterial counts on post- and pre-prostatic massage urines

For answers see over

A.16.7 a. F—Threads in urine may consist of mucus only and may not contain any inflammatory cells.

b. T—Chronic NGU may reflect underlying prostatitis.

c. T—The past history of untreated (for 3 weeks) gonorrhoea should make it mandatory to exclude a urethral stricture. Rarely other renal tract abnormalities will underlie chronic NGU (e.g. bladder stones).

d. T—Meatal warts are a rare but easy to diagnose cause of chronic NGU. Everting the urethral meatus will display these.

e. F—He should be investigated for *T. vaginalis* first — if positive, he *and* his partner should be treated.

f. F—Squeezing the penis and urethra may cause a traumatic urethritis. The patient should be told to stop such activity altogether.

g. T—This may reveal bacterial prostatitis that fails to show up on a mid-stream urine specimen.

Q.16.8 Patricia, who is 21, tells you weepily that ever since she had primary genital herpes she has had recurrent vulval sores present for a few days after intercourse. Apparently, these develop at intercourse, but cultures taken from the ulcers, which are at the fourchette, 3 days later show that herpes simplex virus is present. She tells you that she no longer enjoys intercourse and in fact dreads it.

How would you manage her in the first place?

a. Ask her if she has symptoms consistent with vaginismus and if she lubricates at intercourse
b. Prescribe diazepam regularly
c. Give her a course of acyclovir tablets to prevent recurrence of herpes
d. See her and her partner for sex therapy
e. Tell her that her ulcers are probably traumatic in origin but that they will become infected with herpes as a secondary phenomenon

Q.16.9 Tony, a 32-year-old male homosexual, has been sexually active since the age of 16. A new junior doctor sees him to take routine tests and finds him to have very long arms and legs, to have an early diastolic murmur and a thoracic kyphosis. He has a past history of early syphilis as well as of arthritis in his knees and back.

Which of the following could account for his heart lesion?

a. Marfan's syndrome
b. Mitral stenosis
c. Syphilitic aortitis
d. Reiter's disease
e. Klinefelter's syndrome

For answers see over

A.16.8 a. T—She is almost certainly causing traumatic ulcers to herself at intercourse by the above process.
b. F—This may lead to dependency and is unnecessary in her case.
c. F—There is no need. The ulcers are probably traumatic in nature and become secondary infected with HSV.
d. T—This is the most important aspect of management. Once there is no vaginismus and lubrication returns, the ulceration will probably cease to occur at intercourse.
e. T

A.16.9 a. T—Marfan's syndrome is a cause of relatively long limbs (compared with trunk) and aortic regurgitation.
b. F—Mitral stenosis does not cause an early diastolic murmur.
c. T—Tertiary syphilitic aortitis may lead to aneurysm formation and hence aortic regurgitation.
d. T—Repeated episodes of Reiter's disease may lead to aortic regurgitation and kyphosis secondary to arthritis.
e. F—This is not a cause of aortic valve disease.

Q.16.10 Susan, an 18-year-old prostitute, uses no contraceptives when having intercourse with her boyfriend but sheaths with clients. However, she tells you that 2½ weeks ago, a sheath broke and that now she has severe lower abdominal pain. She thinks the pain could be due to the irritable bowel syndrome she has been told she has, but also feels it may be due to where a seat belt 'caught' her when involved in a minor road accident a week ago.

She is nervous and bimanual examination shows bilateral cervical excitation pain worse on the left. There are no abdominal or adnexal masses but guarding over the left iliac fossa with no rebound tenderness is present. Direct monoclonal slides for *Chlamydia trachomatis* and the gonococcus are both negative.

How would you manage her case?

a. Give her a course of doxycycline for a week and tell her to come back then
b. Prescribe an antispasmodic agent
c. Arrange to see her boyfriend, assess his health and then reassess her
d. Exclude pregnancy as a cause for her symptoms
e. Arrange for a laporascopic examination of her pelvis
f. Treat her for pelvic inflammatory disease (PID)
g. Give her compound codeine for the seat belt injury

For answers see over

A.16.10 a. F—What would the doxycycline be given for? If it was thought that PID was present, metronidazole should be added. However, treatment ought to follow diagnosis which is not established yet.

b. F—It would be dangerous to assume her symptoms are due to colic — either gut or uterine.

c. F—The boyfriend might tell you if she had gonorrhoea or *C. trachomatis* via his positive tests. This is unlikely, however, as her tests are negative. The clinical diagnosis, i.e. whether an ectopic pregnancy or PID, is the pressing question here.

d. T—This may be done by looking for β-human chorionic gonadotrophin in urine where appropriate or by ultrasound scan of the pelvis.

e. T—Laparoscopy. Both d) and e) would be done to exclude ectopic pregnancy.

f. F—Treatment prior to diagnosis is malpractice.

g. F—This may be the diagnosis but PID and ectopic pregnancy should be excluded first.

Q.16.11 A homosexual man attends the clinic for routine tests. During the interview with the doctor the patient mentions that within the next few weeks he will be having several teeth extracted in the hospital dental department. As the patient has always practiced passive anal intercourse with casual partners, the doctor felt that an HIV antibody test should be taken, with a view that should the test prove positive, the patient could inform the dental staff to enable them to take the necessary precautions.

On hearing this, the patient declined the test saying that he knew someone else who informed his dentist that he was HIV antibody positive and was refused dental treatment. The patient added that he did not want anyone apart from the clinic staff and friends to know he was homosexual.

What would you do?

a. Take sufficient blood for syphilis and HIV test without informing the patient
b. Inform the dental department without the patient's consent that they have a 'high-risk' patient
c. Give the patient's name to the dental department and suggest that they refuse to do treatment unless the patient has an HIV blood test
d. Suggest to the dental department that they should test all men for HIV before treatment
e. Explain to the patient that there is no need for HIV antibody testing, but that he should seek a dental practice where known HIV antibody positive patients are handled confidentially and safely

For answers see over

A.16.11 a. F
b. F
c. F
d. F
e. T

Q.16.12 Fortune is with you! You have been asked to become Chief Medical Officer of a central African republic at a salary of $55 000/year. However, the government there is very concerned about the high prevalence of gonorrhoea in the country. Solve it, they tell you, and your salary will be raised to $100 000 per year. Fail and you get the sack.

Which of the following would you implement:

a. Do a survey of the prevalence of gonorrhoea among prostitutes in the cities, ordinary urban dwellers and rural dwellers
b. Educate prostitutes, school children, university students and those at technical colleges about VD
c. Start a mass campaign aimed at blanket treatment of the whole population (this has been done in the past in Greenland)
d. Assess the gonococci found in vitro, i.e. their resistance type and antibiotic sensitivity
e. Make it legally binding to attend a VD clinic if a patient is named as a "gonorrhoea partner".

For answers see over

A.16.12 a. T—Should be set in motion as soon as possible.
b. T—See a) above.
c. F—This type of mass treatment in the past has been unsuccessful in eradicating of infection. In a sexually promiscuous population, only a few people who escape through the net will be enough to ensure continuation of the epidemic.
d. T—See a) above.
e. F—The United Kingdom answer to this question is "false". Legally naming the contact will serve only to drive patients with gonorrhoea away from reliable and reputable sources of treatment.

References

General References

Holmes KK, Mardh PA, Sparling PF, Weisner PJ (1984) Sexually transmitted diseases. McGraw-Hill, New York

Oriel JD, Harris JRW (1986) Recent advances in sexually transmitted diseases, 3. Churchill Livingstone, Edinburgh

Various authors (1980) Disorders caused by biological and environmental agents. In: Isselbacher et al. (eds) Harrison: principles of internal medicine. McGraw-Hill, New York, pp 539–990

Bacterial Vaginosis

Anonymous (1981) Vaginitis revisited Br Med J 283: 745–746

Easmon CSF (1986) Bacterial vaginosis. In: Oriel JD, Harris JRW (eds) Recent advances in sexually transmitted diseases, 3, Churchill Livingstone, Edinburgh

Chlamydial Disease

Darougar S (ed) (1983) Chlamydial disease Br Med Bull 39: 107–203

Oriel JD, Ridgway GL (1982) Genital infection by *Chlamydia trachomatis*. Arnold, London

Taylor-Robinson D, Thomas BJ (1980) The role of *Chlamydia trachomatis* in genital tract and associated diseases. J Clin Path 33: 205–233

Colposcopy

Cartier R (1977) Practical colposcopy. Karger, Basel

Walker PG, Singer A, Dyson JL, Shah KV, Wilters J, Coleman DV (1983) Colposcopy in the diagnosis of papillomavirus infection of the uterine cervix. BJ Obstet Gynaecol 90: 1082–1086

Warts

Campion MJ, Singer A, Clarkson PK, McLance DJ (1985) Increased risk of cervical neoplasia in the consorts of men with penile condyloma acuminata. Lancet I: 943–945

Editorial (1985) Genital warts, human papillomavirus and cervical cancer. Lancet II: 1045–1046

Singer A, Walker PG, McLance DJ (1984) Genital wart virus infection: nuisance or potentially lethal? Br Med J 1984: 288: 735–737

Gonorrhoea

Holmes KK, Mardh PA, Sparling PF, Weisner PJ (1984) Sexually transmitted diseases. McGraw-Hill, New York, Chaps 19, 21

Proctitis

Goldmeier D (1985) Proctitis. In: clinical problems in sexually transmitted diseases. Martinus Nijhoff, Dordrecht, pp 238–284

Hepatitis

Hoofnagle JH (1981) Serological markers of hepatitis B virus infection. Ann Rev Med 32: 1–11

Dienstag JL, Wands JR, Koff RS (1980) Acute hepatitis. In: Isselbacher KJ, Adams RD, Braunwald E, Petersdorf RS, Wilson JD (eds) Principles of internal medicine. McGraw-Hill, New York, pp 1459–1470

Feinstone SM, Hoofnagle JH (1984) Non A, maybe B hepatitis. New Engl J Med 311: 185–188

Thomas HC (1985) The delta antigen comes of age. Gut 26: 1–3

Genital Herpes

Corey L, Holmes KK (1983) Genital herpes simplex virus infections. Current concepts in diagnosis, therapy and prevention. Ann Int Med 98: 973–983

Mindel A, Faherty A, Hindley D, Weller IVD, Sutherland S, Fiddian AP, Adler MW (1984) Prophylactic oral Acyclovir in recurrent genital herpes. Lancet ii: 57–59

Aids and Immunology

Pinching AJ (1985) Clinical aspects of AIDS and other HTLV III related conditions. In: Oriel JD (ed) Recent advances in sexually transmitted diseases, 3. Churchill Livingstone, Edinburgh

Pinching AJ, Weiss RA (to be published) AIDS and the spectrum of HTLV III/LAV infection I. In: Richter GW, Epstein MA (eds) International review of experimental pathology, vol 28

Seligmann M, Chess L, Fahey JL, Fauci AS, Lachmann PJ, L'age-Stehr J, Ngu J, Pinching AJ, Rosen FS, Spira TJ, Wybran J (1984) AIDS — an immunologic re-evaluation. N Engl J Med 311: 1286–1292

Roitt IM, Brostoff J, Male DK (eds) (1985) Immunology. Churchill Livingstone, Edinburgh

Pelvic Inflammatory Disease

Mardh PA (1980) An overview of infectious agents of salpingitis, their biology and recent advances in methods of detection. Am J Obstet Gynecol 138: 933–951

Jacobson L, Westrom L (1969) Objectivised diagnosis of acute PID. Am J Obstet Gynecol 105: 1088–1098

Prostatitis

Kreiger JN (1984), Prostatitis syndromes: pathophysiology, differential diagnosis and treatment, Sex Trans Dis 11: 100–113

Psychosexual

Bancroft J (1985) Human sexuality and its problems. Churchill Livingstone, Edinburgh

Frost DP (1985) Recognition of hypochondriasis in a clinic for sexually transmitted diseases. Genito Med 61: 133–137

Syphilis

King A, Nicol C, Rodin P (1980) Venereal diseases, 4th edn. Balliere Tindall, London pp 1–171

GPSR Compliance

The European Union's (EU) General Product Safety Regulation (GPSR) is a set of rules that requires consumer products to be safe and our obligations to ensure this.

If you have any concerns about our products, you can contact us on ProductSafety@springernature.com

In case Publisher is established outside the EU, the EU authorized representative is:

Springer Nature Customer Service Center GmbH
Europaplatz 3
69115 Heidelberg, Germany

Batch number: 09635029

Printed by Printforce, the Netherlands